L. P. Meredith

The Teeth and How to Save Them

L. P. Meredith

The Teeth and How to Save Them

ISBN/EAN: 9783337314842

Printed in Europe, USA, Canada, Australia, Japan

Cover: Foto ©Lupo / pixelio.de

More available books at **www.hansebooks.com**

THE TEETH

AND

HOW TO SAVE THEM.

BY

L. P. MEREDITH, M.D., D.D.S.

"*Tibi seris, tibi metis.*"

PHILADELPHIA:
J. B. LIPPINCOTT & CO.
1871.

CONTENTS.

	Page.
Preface	7
Introductory Chapter	9
History of Dentistry	13
Food in Relation to the Teeth	21
Origin and Formation of the Teeth	34
Eruption of the Temporary Teeth	40
The Troubles of First Dentition	43
Lancing the Gums During First Dentition	49
Preservation of Temporary Teeth	55
The Permanent Teeth	59
The Troubles of Second Dentition	64
Description of the Permanent Teeth	66
Irregularity of the Teeth	71
Dental Caries, or Decay	77
Filling, or Plugging	93
Mallet Filling	122
The File	125
Separating	127
Coffer Dam Rubber	130
Bleaching the Teeth	131
Salivary Calculus, or Tartar	133
Odontalgia, or Toothache	138
Miscellaneous Diseases	167
Third Dentition	183
Supernumerary Teeth	186
United Teeth	188

	Page.
Extracting	189
Anæsthesia	200
Nitrous Oxide Gas.	203
Dentifrices, Brushes, etc	226
Tobacco.	229
Artificial Teeth	233
Defects of the Palate	256
Quackery	258
Index	269

PREFACE.

THE profession of DENTISTRY after a period of infancy, longer, perhaps, than that of any other profession, dating from the earliest history of man to within a comparatively recent day, has taken the prominent position that it now occupies. Beginning its strife for eminence cotemporaneously with the science of medicine, it has been compelled for centuries to remain almost unnoticed, while its more fortunate and more needed brother has ever pressed forward into the foremost ranks of notice and honor.

But its seclusion has not been passed in idleness; while waiting in silence and abiding its time, it has been gathering the crumbs that have fallen from the tables of knowledge, and to-day, when the urgent need of humanity calls it forth, it comes bearing its unlimited gatherings from the treasures of Philosophy, Chemistry, Medicine and Art, and claiming equal right to contribute to the wants of the suffering race.

But while the profession of DENTISTRY stands thus ready and willing to bestow its favors upon all who desire them, the fact is nevertheless too evident that few, comparatively, avail themselves of their opportunity.

Then, again, many who profess a desire for its services are ushered in at the wrong door by the seductive wiles of empiricism, and obtain instructions so corrupted and so abused by unscientific handling, that injury follows more often than benefit.

The great cause of the success of Charlatanism is, that the *true profession* has stood back too much on its dignity, and has waited to be sought rather than to seek; however well it deserves this mark of respect, it is nevertheless true that it has not been properly appreciated because the *people* have been denied the right kind of information.

It is with the intention, therefore, of opening the doors of dental knowledge to the people; of explaining its fundamental principles to the best of his moderate ability, and of giving such suggestions and information relative to its uses and abuses as may awaken a better appreciation, that the author, a humble votary of DENTISTRY, offers this little volume to the public.

CINCINNATI, O., July, 1871.

INTRODUCTORY CHAPTER.

IT has often been a matter of wonder to me that many books of the nature of this have not been written. Numerous subjects of far less importance than the human teeth have been again and again treated of in books intended for domestic use. People have been instructed how to take care of their flowers, trees and gardens; their bees, birds and cattle; their hair, eyes and complexion. Volume after volume of "domestic medicine" has been published. In short, nearly every subject, excepting dentistry, that has been considered of importance to the comfort, well-being or profit of mankind, has been brought by means of books into the family circle for familiar contemplation. This is not because the profession of dentistry has not the material from which to furnish such instruction. Dental colleges are flourishing all over the land; associations are meeting almost daily, where the thousands of their members are engaged in discussing subjects of infinite interest to themselves and the people; standard dental works occupy their places in the library of the practitioner, while the dental journals, containing the thoughts and experience of the brightest lights in the profession, are so numerous and so replete with information, that no one can find time or opportunity to read them all. But from this great storehouse of knowledge the dentists alone procure instruction; the public is not at all educated in proportion to the advancement of the profession.

Considering these facts, may I not then be excused for endeavoring, even in my imperfect way, to bridge over this stream of ignorance that lies between the profession and the masses?

In undertaking this labor, I am considerably perplexed at the start in deciding how to condense the greatest amount of useful matter in the smallest possible compass; for such condensation is necessary in order not to exceed the limits of an ordinary sized volume.

If I should attempt to describe all of the anatomy of the teeth and surrounding parts—the bones, muscles, tissues, arteries, veins, nerves, glands, etc.—all of which would be necessary to give a *complete* idea of the anatomical relations, those things alone would take up a good-sized volume. The same might be said if I should propose to speak particularly of the physiological action of these different parts; the uses and repair of the osseous portions; the actions of the muscles; the conveyance of nutritive material through the arterial system, and the removal of waste through the veins and absorbents; the secretions of the salivary and mucous glands, and the direct and sympathetic pain and other nervous impressions occurring in abnormal conditions. All of these subjects and various points in chemistry, philosophy and medicine would have to be explained in order to convey anything like *thorough* instruction in dental knowledge.

While it would be impossible to treat of these subjects in the present work, yet the information alluded to can be readily and pleasantly acquired by any one who so wishes, upon reference to one or more of the dental text-books of the present time.

With these hints as to the sources and usefulness of a good general dental education, and with an earnest wish that my readers may have their appreciation awakened sufficiently to spend a few leisure hours in acquiring such knowledge, I proceed to the accomplishment of my design, which is to lay before my readers something of the history of dentistry; the origin, formation and eruption of the teeth; the methods of securing their regular arrangement and healthy constitution; the causes of the diseases of the teeth and mouth, and their prevention and cure, and the restoration by artificial appliances of parts that have been lost by disease, accident or negligence.

In the consideration of these and various incidental topics calculated to promote the advancement of dental knowledge among the people, my efforts shall be applied.

That the state of the times requires earnest and successful labors in this direction, we have but to look around us to see. Thousands of people, tolerably well-informed on other subjects, patronize the dentist only to have teeth *extracted*, and believe *filling* to be injurious and promotive of decay. With numbers to *clean* the teeth is the *exception* and not the *rule;* tartar and decomposing food thus accumulating and injuring the gums and teeth, vitiating the saliva, producing impure breath, impure blood, dyspepsia, and ills without number. Thousands of sickly parents are begetting sickly children with sickly teeth, and instead of feeding them with such food as is calculated to counterbalance the inherited predisposition, are doing just the opposite. And thousands more through fear of a little discomfort in the dental chair, or through pecuniary closeness, are permitting themselves to be lulled into sweet oblivion by anæsthetic influence, and sacrifice their own *nature's* teeth for the "beautiful teeth" of the cheap charlatan.

If these and many other evils connected with the times do not call for reformation, then indeed is the mission of the dentist a mistaken one.

In offering this volume as a companion for the household, I would beg leave to state that the teachings herein contained are not mere dogmas of my own, but are truths deduced, either from my actual experience or from the best authorities, and may, therefore, be taken as reliable guides as far as the present status of dental science is concerned.

HISTORY OF DENTISTRY.

IN tracing any business, art or profession, back to its beginning, one naturally turns to the Old Testament to see what is recorded in its truthful pages in reference to it. But concerning the subject of dentistry, the data are so few that we are led to believe the teeth, in those days, were remarkably good, and subject to no disease of sufficient moment to call into life a special profession for their treatment. There is no doubt that the teeth were appreciated on account of their service and adornment, and that their loss was considered a serious misfortune; for in the Mosaic law we find: "If a man smite out his manservant's tooth or his maid-servant's tooth, he shall *let him go free* for his tooth's sake." Then in Solomon's Song, setting forth the graces of the Church in the most beautiful figures, we see: "Thy teeth are like a flock of sheep that are even shorn, which came up from the washing; whereof every one beareth twins, and there is not one barren among them." It does not take much stretch of the imagination to see the allusion to the *evenness*, the *whiteness*, the *two of each kind*, the *presence of all*, which are embodied in a beautiful set of teeth to-day as well as then. That the effects of certain chemical agents were known in those days, we conclude from the passage in Proverbs: "As vinegar to the teeth, and as smoke to the eyes, so is the sluggard to them that send him." And again, in Jeremiah: "Every man that eateth the sour grape, his teeth shall be set on edge."

In enforcing the penalty of the law, "Eye for eye, tooth for tooth," it is probable that if the loss of the complainant was not atoned for by some pecuniary satisfaction, it was the duty of some officer to extract a similar tooth from the offender, and he was certainly a *dentist* for the time being.

Although the explanations of the commentaries are so unsatisfactory concerning the exclamation of Job in his groanings: "I am escaped with the skin of my teeth;" yet it hardly seems possible that he could have been acquainted with their delicate anatomy. It seems strange, however, that his language should anticipate the discovery, more than three thousand years later, of the "cuticle of the enamel." Any one waggishly inclined might force a resemblance between Job and the untutored quack of modern times, when he said, alluding to his past days of prosperity: "And I brake the jaws of the wicked, and plucked the spoil out of his teeth."

When we come, however, to search the annals of profane history, we do not find such a scanty supply of material connected with the profession of dentistry; but the truths are so few and so mixed up with ignorance and superstition, that it is a matter of curiosity rather than of benefit to refer to them. From the writings of Herodotus (about 450 B. C.), we learn that the treatment of the teeth constituted a separate branch of practice among the Egyptians, and the truth of this is corroborated by the testimony of the celebrated Giovanni Belzoni, noted for his discoveries in Egypt. He informs us that in the ancient tombs artificial teeth of ivory and wood were found, some fastened on gold plates. Gold fillings, also, have been found in the teeth of mummies. Horace, Ovid, and other ancient poets allude to artificial teeth. In those early days charms and amulets were employed for the relief of the toothache, and little knowledge appeared to exist concerning its causes, as we would judge from such teachings as that offered by Aretœus, a Greek physician of the first century, who gave it as his learned opinion that "the cause of toothache was known only to God." Galen, in the second century, considered that the teeth possessed the power of taste as well as the tongue, on account of the nerves that entered their roots. Leaping over a space of about fourteen hundred years to the time of the eminent Lord Bacon (1560 to 1626 A. D.), we are disappointed in any hopes of considerable advancement of dental knowledge; which, if existing, we might reasonably expect to see in one of such versatile genius, and so learned in the literature of all nations. He appears to have devoted much attention to the teeth, and says that the points to be considered regarding them are: "The preserving of them; the keeping of them white; the drawing of them with the least pain; the staying and easing of the toothache; the binding in of artificial teeth, and the great one of restoring teeth in old age."

In a book, published not much later, "The Works of that Learned and Renowned Doctor Lazarus Riverius, sometimes Councillor and Physitian to the King of France," we find such instructions as the following: Charles Piso being troubled with the toothache many days, "half an hour after he had taken purging medicine, vomited up above a pint of clear water with such success that ten years after he was never troubled with it." He was led to believe that a surplus of some humor in the body was the cause of it, because he observed that persons that "have the toothache do continually *spet*."

Further on, Riverius mentions *worms* in the cavity of decay as one of the causes of toothache and says: "If worms are the cause of pain it will be intermitting, coming and going often, and sometimes the motion of the worm will be felt." Afterward he judiciously prescribes a bitter application to kill the worms. Again we read: "And because the small veins by which nourishment is carried to the teeth do run by the ears, you may put medicine into them for the cure of toothache." He then gives some kind advice to the patients, whose interest he has so much at heart, in case that they are obliged to present a tooth for extraction to some of the skillful operators of the day: "And the Chirurgeon is to be admonished that he pull it not out violently at one pull, lest the brain be too much shaken and the jaw-bone broken, from whence comes a great flux of blood, a *feaver* and sometimes *death*." After proposing different remedies for the toothache, he says: "But the leaf of Elleboraster rubbed upon the tooth is best; but you must not touch the others, lest they also fall out."

In the experiment of Leuwenhoeck, in 1678, we perceive an important step toward the correct anatomy of the teeth. He drew out one of his own teeth for observation, and discovered with the aid of his glass that "the whole tooth was made up of very small, straight and transparent pipes. 600 or 700 of these pipes put together exceed not the thickness of one hair of a man's beard." But Dr. Hugh Todd, a well educated man of the same times, in examining a disinterred skeleton twenty-two feet long, at Corbridge, on the Tyne, did not know whether the teeth, three or four inches in compass, were *human* or not. About a hundred years later than this, which brings us to the door of the nineteenth century, the renowned Hufeland, in the "*Art of Prolonging Life*," gave this advice: "As soon as you observe that a tooth is decayed, have it immediately pulled out, otherwise it will infect the rest." At the beginning of the nineteenth century there was, comparatively speaking, but little diffusion of dental knowledge, even among professional men; although from the labors of such men as Fallopius and Eustachius, of Italy, and Paré, of France, in the sixteenth century; Martin, in the seventeenth; Fauchard and Bourdet, of France, in the middle of the eighteenth century, and Hunter and Fox, of England, some years later; there had resulted such an accumulation of general principles and such a sifting of truth from error, that a sure foundation stone was laid upon which to erect the imposing structure of the present times.

It is not worth while to weary the reader with the successive steps in the advancement of dental science, when once the hindrances being removed from its path, it made its rapid strides toward perfection. It is its present condition that most interests us, and of this it is the object of the subsequent pages of this work to treat.

It may not be amiss, however, to give some general idea of the work that has been accomplished in different departments within a little more than half a century. Incorruptible porcelain artificial teeth have taken the place of transplanted human teeth and teeth carved from those of sheep and other animals, and from bone and ivory. Pure gold in various forms, unchangeable and so admirably adapted for the preservation of decayed teeth, by filling, has superseded the inferior and less durable metals. Artificial teeth on plates secured by atmospheric pressure have done away with the old methods of fastening them by ligatures, clasps and springs. Aching teeth that a few years ago used to be lost, almost invariably, are now often saved and made permanently useful. The extraction of teeth that used to be an operation of so much pain to all and agony to many, is now rendered almost pleasant by means of anæsthetics. Fissures and openings into the palate, caused by disease and wounds, that used so much to interfere with speech and deglutition as to make life miserable, are now remedied to such an extent as to cause but little inconvenience. A number of dental colleges has been established, having centered in them all the talent and facilities to educate those choosing the dental profession, in a manner that a lifetime of practice would scarcely equal. Dental magazines, filled with all of the extracts from the fields of science and art that can in any way benefit the dentist and better prepare him to practice his profession, have multiplied to a number almost too great for perusal. Dental societies, to the profession, have almost become as prayer-meetings to the churches. The number of dentists in the United States alone has increased from less than a dozen, in 1800, to more than 10,000; while there is not a suffering mortal in the smallest village anywhere in the civilized world that does not have more or less convenient access to some one devoted to the practice of dentistry. Of course *very many* of these are uneducated men and unworthy of the name of dentists in the true acceptation of the word; but if the people can be educated up to the point of being able to discern what ought to be the acquirements of the dentist, and of refusing their patronage to charlatans—thus compelling them to enlighten themselves—then will the dental profession have shaken off its last reproach.

FOOD IN RELATION TO THE TEETH.

IF the builders of a house are supplied with poor brick and poor stone, bad timber and bad mortar, the workmen, no matter how skillful they are, can erect nothing but a weak and insubstantial edifice. So Nature, in building the human fabric, approaches perfection more or less nearly, according to the materials furnished. From the food taken into the body are all the different parts of that body formed and maintained. If the food eaten during the time of formation is deficient in certain constituents essential to different parts, those portions are imperfectly organized and rendered incapable of fulfilling the objects of their creation.

Of the sixty-four elements to which all the various substances in the world have been reduced, fourteen enter into the composition of the human organism. Chemical analysis has shown these to be carbon, nitrogen, hydrogen, oxygen, phosphorus, calcium, sulphur, fluorine, chlorine, sodium, iron, potassium, magnesium and silicon. These are introduced by solid food, liquids and air into the system, and are found there in the form of proximate principles or substances composed of two or more ultimate elements, as shown in the following examples:

WATER, composed of hydrogen and oxygen, is found in all the solids and fluids of the body and constitutes about three-fourths of it by weight.

CHLORIDE OF SODIUM (COMMON SALT) is composed of chlorine and sodium, and is detected in all parts of the body, except the enamel of the teeth.

PHOSPHATE OF LIME, formed of phosphorus, oxygen and calcium, is the principal ingredient in the earthy matter of the bones.

FATS, composed of carbon, hydrogen and oxygen.

Besides these are found, albumen fibrin, osteine, globuline, carbonate of lime, fluoride of calcium, phosphates of soda, potash and magnesia, sulphate and carbonate of soda, peroxide of iron, silica and other proximate principles. Chemical analysis again has shown just what articles of food contain these different constituents. Physiology has classified alimentary substances under three principal heads: those which produce fat and furnish heat to the body; those which supply muscle, etc.; and those which supply bone, brain and nerves. The body can not be sustained by any *one* of these classes. As Dr. Dalton says in his Treatise on Human Physiology: " In order that the animal tissues and fluids remain in a healthy condition and take their proper part in the functions of life, they must be supplied with all the ingredients necessary to their constitution, and a man may be starved to death at last by depriving him of chloride of sodium or phosphate of lime just as surely, though not so rapidly, as if he were deprived of albumen or oil."

It will not be in accordance with the design of this work to enter into a minute consideration of the different alimentary principles and their relation to the well-being of the body, however closely this subject may be connected with the condition of the mouth as a part of the whole, or with the support of health and vital power during the process of dentition; but there are a few points that demand some attention.

PHOSPHATE OF LIME.

This substance is of great interest to us as regards the teeth. It constitutes the greater portion of them, and is what gives them their extreme hardness. The importance of phosphate of lime to the osseous structure is well proven by the oft-tried experiment of placing a bone in dilute muriatic acid, when the phosphate is dissolved, and the animal matter remaining behind, and retaining the form of the bone, becomes so pliable that it can be bent in any direction, or even tied in a knot. Other earthy matters enter into the construction of the teeth, but they are in small quantities and not sufficient to preserve their integrity. Nature forms the teeth of such material as is present in the blood. If from any cause there is a deficient supply of the phosphate, they are more or less imperfectly constructed, and come forth either with fissures. or so soft in structure as to be soon affected by the various causes of decay.

Parallel instances in the operations of nature are seen in the softening of the bones (osteomalacia) of adults, and the rickets of children, diseases caused by a deficiency of the phosphate of lime. The same is seen in the formation of the egg, the yolk of which passes through the oviduct having albuminous substance secreted around it, then a firm fibrous covering, and finally in the last part of the oviduct has calcareous salts crystallized in the substance of the fibrous membrane, forming the shell. If the fowl is denied access to material for shell the eggs are laid without them. Now there is no doubt that the bad teeth of the youth of the present day are attributable more to the imperfect supply of phosphate of lime, than to any other cause. This insufficiency exists before birth in the blood of the mother, and after birth in the milk and food given to the child. In this connection the bread, pastry, cake, etc., so much in use and made of superfine flour, have received more blame than anything else.

The distribution of the elements in wheat answers the wants of the human system better than any other grain; but in the ordinary method of preparing, it is ascertained that the most essential constituents are removed. The outer portions of the grain containing the material for bone, muscle and brain, being tenacious and flaky, are mostly sifted off, leaving hardly anything in the flour but starch. Many parents eat no other kind of flour than this, and many children after weaning are almost brought up on such flour, with sugar and butter added. Add to this cause the degenerated physical condition of the mother of the present times, inherited imperfections, unhealthy milk, the cultivated taste for fancy dishes, and the wonder is, not that children have bad teeth, but that they have any teeth at all. It is stated that "an insufficient supply of phosphate of lime is supposed to account for the well known fact that women, when pregnant, suffer unduly from toothache, the tooth substance of the mother being attacked in order to supply material for that of the offspring." Bran contains fourteen times as much material for bone and muscle as fine flour does; therefore the use of unbolted flour and cracked wheat is indicated for both mother and child. The condition of the teeth is not bettered to any appreciable extent by food taken into the system after they are formed; so the time to furnish the necessary constituents is while they are developing.

If the first set is poor, let it be the care that the second shall not be so. Young children should not be allowed to acquire a taste solely for white bread, pastry, butter, sugar and confectioneries, but they should be accustomed to use broiled beefsteak and the gravy therefrom, other meats, barley, oatmeal, vegetables, sweet potatoes especially, eggs, and allowed to drink plenty of pure milk; or when nursing and too young to take these things, the mother should be plentifully supplied with them. If some of these articles should not agree with the child others should be tried. Mucilage of rice has often been recommended as being soothing, somewhat constipating, and containing a useful quantity of phosphate of lime in solution. It is made by boiling rice well in a surplus of water.

MILK.

Through the wisdom of the Creator, who always intends in his works that the means shall be adequate to the end, the healthy human milk from the healthy mother is sufficient for all the requirements of the infant, at least until the teeth begin to come, the very appearance of which seems to indicate that the child needs, in addition to the mother's supply, some solid food which requires mastication. In the human milk are found casein, the albuminous substance for the formation of muscle; sugar and butter for heat and fat; and mineral matter for bones, teeth, etc. But for many reasons, which it is not worth while to mention here, it is a lamentable truth that a great number of the mothers of the present times are not able to supply their children with milk of the proper quality or in sufficient quantity.

This makes it necessary to seek a supply from some other source; and it is this compulsory change, occurring at a time when the delicate constitution of the child will bear so little tampering with, that causes a large share of the mortality of infancy. A wet-nurse is without doubt the best substitute, if a suitable one can be obtained, but it is seldom indeed that such a one can be secured. The case is so urgent and the time for inquiry into the history of the nurse is so short, that generally the first one that offers is taken, and it is more a matter of chance than choice. The nurse's age should not be far from that of the mother, and her confinement should have taken place at about the same time; she should be in good health, with no inherited or other constitutional disease lurking in her system; her moral conduct during the time of her services should be above reproach; she should be of kind disposition and should be willing to yield to sensible dictation in regard to her cleanliness, exercise, diet, etc. How rarely all of these things can be expected from one who gives her services for wages to the highest bidder, with no parental love for the little being, not her own, at her breast, can be imagined. Sudden emotions, as anger and fear, sometimes produce diarrhœa, convulsions, etc., in the infant. Salivation may occur from the milk of a nurse who is under the influence of mercury; and all unhealthy conditions of the milk more or less affect the child.

Unless every serious doubt could be dismissed from the mind of the parent, I would have no hesitation in advising bottle-feeding in preference to the wet-nurse. But here also, especially in cities, great difficulties are encountered. Very little *pure* milk can be obtained in spite of municipal regulations and official inspection. The art of milk adulteration has become a science almost. The most common method is to remove a portion of the cream and add water; and then, to improve the color of the impoverished milk, different substances are mixed with it. Observation of the amount of cream furnished by a small quantity of milk, compared with some known to be pure, is the best method of detecting this fraud. Gum, flour, starch, chalk and emulsion of sheep's brains, are other substances used for adulteration. The granules of starch can be detected by the microscope; or solution of iodine will turn them blue. Chalk will settle to the bottom of the vessel, and may be recognized by muriatic acid causing it to effervesce. Shreds of nerve substance from the brain may be detected by the microscope. Milk is often furnished that is derived from an unhealthy or improperly fed animal; it is generally characterized by some unnatural odor or taste, or by its containing pus or mucus. Considering the great interest at stake, it is certainly a duty to have milk that is offered for the sustenance of the child, and represented to be pure, occasionally examined by a practical chemist. Supposing, however, that after due care, pure milk from a healthy cow is secured, it must be remembered that it is richer in casein, butter and phosphates than human milk, but poorer in sugar; therefore it should be diluted with about one-third water and have a little sugar added. Asses' milk is much better than cow's milk if it can be procured. Two parts of it should be added to one part of cow's milk. An artificial asses' milk is made by adding two ounces of sugar of milk, or unmedicated homœopathic globules, to a pint of skimmed cow's milk. Arrowroot, flour and other starch pastes, with sugar and butter, should not alone be employed to sustain the child, as often done. Starch, butter and sugar give fat and make it plump and round, but they don't furnish a fibre of muscle or a granule of bone or tooth substance.

SUGAR.

No article of food is mentioned, in reference to effects upon the teeth after their eruption, as frequently as sugar. The popular belief is that it causes decay. If a child's temporary teeth break down at an early age from imperfect organization, lack of cleanliness or what not, the parent attributes it to sugar. If the permanent teeth, from the before mentioned causes, or from irregular position, or lack of understanding in their management, are presented to the dentist gone almost beyond remedy at an age when they should be perfect, the parent begins with a tirade against sugar. In short, sugar is the "scapegoat" for nearly all the ignorance and negligence concerning the teeth and their requirements. It is one of that class of words so often used by habit, more than through any knowledge of their signification, sounding well but meaning nothing, like "cold" and "neuralgia." A person has the toothache and he ventures the opinion that it is caused by "cold;" the listener knowingly nods his head in assent, yet neither of them knows anything about *how* cold produces change in the circulation of a part, or how that change causes irritation of the nerves; and, in the majority of instances, "cold" is innocent of the charge. If one has an attack of sharp, flitting pain that he can not at once trace to its origin, he calls it "neuralgia," and he is right about once in a hundred times. Nineteen out of twenty that abuse sugar as the agent of so much mischief, can not give one reason for its producing such effects. This prejudice against sugar originated in olden times, and has been handed down to posterity, with no more testimony in substantiation of the charge then, than now. In *Paul Heintzner's Travels*, 1598, Queen Elizabeth is said to have "her teeth black from eating too much sugar." I don't doubt from what history says of her that her teeth were bad, but I suppose it was only a case of dental caries, no worse than we see nowadays in ladies that are not queens. Lord Bacon, in his discourse in praise of the Queen, describes her gait, hair, voice, eyes, etc., but keeps silent in regard to her *teeth*, from which I infer that the appearance of her mouth was not as prepossessing as it ought to be in a lady who supported so much style. But my respect for royalty has caused me to digress. Let us see what evidence can be found in favor of sugar. History tells us that "Henry, Duke of Beaufort, who died about 1702, ate nearly a pound of sugar daily for forty years. He died of fever in the seventieth year of his age. He was never troubled with cough, his teeth were firm, and all his viscera were found, after death, quite sound." In Cleland's Institutes of Health, Mallory is described as a great lover and eater of sugar, and is said to have lived to be about one hundred years of age, and to have had good teeth until fourscore, when he cut a new set.

Sir John Sinclair, in his work on Health and Longevity, repeats what was affirmed by Dr. Slare, in the latter part of the seventeenth century, that his grandfather, who lived to be one hundred years old, had all his teeth strong and firm at eighty; that he remained in good health and strength till his death, and died in consequence of fullness of blood. These circumstances were attributed by Dr. Slare to the *frequent use of sugar*, of which his grandfather was a great eater, taking it on his bread and butter, in ale and beer, and adding it to all the sauces used on his meats. These are a few of the many instances furnished by men of repute to establish the fact that *sugar is not injurious to the teeth*. The negroes of sugar countries are remarkable for their white and sound teeth, although they eat great quantities of sugar, and grow fat on it during the season for making it. Teeth have been immersed for a year or more in a syrup of sugar and water, and when taken out have not been affected in the least degree. Now, a few words to show that saccharine matter as food is absolutely necessary for the growing child. The proportion of phosphate of lime required by the child is greater than in the adult, for, in the first instance, the bones are increasing in size, while in the adult they only have to be maintained. The lactic acid, that is formed from the sugar, dissolves the phosphate of lime in other articles of food, and thus prepares it to readily enter the circulation.

Then, again, circulation and respiration being more active in the growing being than in one who has ceased to grow, some especial food is required to be consumed in the lungs, and protect the parts already organized from the action of oxygen. Children have an instinctive desire for some such food; the colder the climate the richer must the substance be in hydrogen and carbon for furnishing heat. Accordingly we would naturally expect that the children in the frigid zone would crave some richer material. Such we find to be the case. Sir Anthony Carlisle says: "In one of those late extravagant voyages to discover a northwest passage, the most northern races of mankind were found to be unacquainted with the taste of sweets, and their infants made very wry faces, and sputtered out sugar with disgust; but the little urchins grinned with ecstasy at the sight of a bit of whale's blubber."

Now, in conclusion, I do not wish to be understood that sugar can not be made a source of evil. Biting into rock and other hard candies is certainly a very reprehensible practice, and will injure a set of teeth as much as cracking nuts with them or biting other hard substances. Then, sugar should not be allowed to the point of producing stomach disturbances and diarrhœa. Sour regurgitations are injurious to the teeth, but no more so when arising from a stomach made sour by too much sugar, than from the same condition caused by any other article of food.

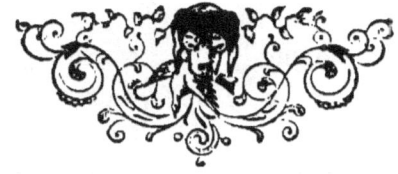

ORIGIN AND FORMATION OF THE TEETH.

THE teeth are generally classed, as regards the method of their formation, with such substances as horn, hair and nails. Being partially external and increasing in size by successive deposits of formative material, there are certainly striking similarities.

Many scientific men have devoted much valuable time to the study of this wonderful process of nature, and, as in every other study connected with minute microscopical examination, their conclusions have been various and conflicting. To mention their different ideas in regard to the growth of the enamel, dentine and cementum, the different membranes from which they are formed, etc., would greatly extend this article, and prove, I fear, very uninteresting to the general reader.

Certainly the most simple and comprehensible explanation I have ever seen, is that given by Dr. Jas. E. Garretson, in his "Diseases and Surgery of the Mouth, Jaws and Associate Parts." And as simplicity is what is desired in the present work, I shall give his thoughts with a few omissions, and possibly some slight alterations. Wherein his opinions conflict with the views of others, he will have to fight his own battles, which he is doubtless able and willing to do. They are certainly reasonable and consistent, and worthy of acceptation until they can be *proven* erroneous.

At the sixth week of intra-uterine existence there is a groove observable in the gums of the fœtus— "lined by a delicate membrane continuous with the mucous membrane, and perhaps a part of it. * * * This membrane, at points corresponding with the position of the future teeth, is elevated into papillæ or little hills. A section through the membrane, over any of the bulbs, exposes a papilla. * * * This papilla is the rudiment of the future tooth, as observation of its development proves. * * * The papilla, thus understood, is seen to lie beneath the mucous membrane, and in this membrane resides a certain amount of elasticity. As the papilla enlarges and projects itself, it becomes inclosed to all the extent possible with this mucous membrane contracted about the body, so as to constitute a sac or cell wall. * * * This sac enveloping the papilla has its continuation, as is seen, necessarily over the sides of the groove; as then this groove enlarges and deepens, and finally envelopes the papilla, it is seen that the body or tooth-germ gets a second sac. * * * At this period, the pulp or original papilla, having attained the size of the tooth it represents, commences the process of the formation of dentine. Before the attainment to full size of the papilla there existed between it and its sac proper a fluid. This fluid is now replaced by a more highly endowed secretion, the work of matured cells. This secretion, deposited against the inner sac, or between it and the pulp, contains the elements of the dentinal structure, is, indeed, the dentine, and deposits layer after layer, supported by and molded into form by the sac. As this deposit intrudes on the pulp, so this body contracts within itself, until, finally, by some law of nature, it stops at that certain point which maintains within the tooth a canal or cavity, and a vascular and nervous pulp to occupy it,—this pulp being the contracted original papilla; the vessels of this papilla being vessels entirely analagous to any one of the ordinary papilla of touch, so supplied and so maintained. Why this secretion, in its organization, should assume the position of the elongated tubular cells which pertains to the structure of dentine, I have, of course, no idea, and it is quite enough for our purpose to say that it is a law of life perhaps never to be comprehended this side of eternity, and the discovery of which would, at any rate, have but little practical signification to us."

[The cause of this tubular structure of the dentine is doubtless a matter more of curiosity than practical interest, but a thought has sometimes suggested itself to me which it may not be amiss to state. Taking as texts the statements of Kölliker, of Würzburg, that "according to their more or less frequent ramification, are the ends of the dentinal canals more or less fine; frequently appearing merely as excessively fine, pale lines, like fibrils of connective tissue," and that "the dental sacs consist of connective tissue in which vessels and nerves are distributed," I would ask if there may not be such connective tissue between the papilla and the sac, which being stretched in lines, while the papilla and the sac are being separated, are fixed in position by the deposition of the dentine. To illustrate, by a homely comparison, let us suppose that two solid substances are placed against each other with a layer of glue between them; before the glue is hardened draw them apart and numerous strings of connection will be seen, and if plaster of Paris is poured in, there will be a solid substance formed full of delicate tubes corresponding with the direction of the partial separation.]

"The formation of the dentine completed, the covering of it with enamel begins, or rather this deposit is, to a degree, coincident with the dentinal formation. Secreted by the same pulp which formed the dentine, the same secretion, some portion of it finds its way into and through the primary sac. As it passes through this sac it is modified, receives new elements, perhaps, which as it is received into the second space, or the space between the first and second caps, and its calcification commences, impresses upon it the arrangement of its particles after the hexagonal order of the enamel. Between the enamel thus formed and the dentine, exists the primary sac;

simply the originally modified mucous membrane which we first saw as overlying the papilla. This membrane continues its existence between these two hard bodies, and receives and modifies for the support of the enamel, the liquor sanguinis sucked out from the dentinal tubules and intertubular structure. It may be called the enamel membrane. It has, of course, been much modified, and it is from it that we receive the impressions of pain when it is exposed by a break in the continuity of the enamel. The growth of the root of the tooth, as far as its dentine is concerned, has precisely the history of the body. It is associated with the pyramidal elongation of the papilla or pulp, which, pushing upward the crown, elongates upon itself the enamel membrane. This elongation, with a greater vascularity and vitality assumed by the membrane as it approaches the basement vessels, modifies again the result obtained by the secretion passing through it from the dentinal pulp, the result being a nearer approach to true bone in the production of cementum. The periodonteum is simply the modified external sac, lost, of course, above the neck as the tooth has emerged through it. * * * About the fourth month (of fœtal life) these papillæ are all in their sacular envelopes, and forming behind the lids of the sacs are little crescentic depressions, called cavities of reserve, lined with mucous membrane and containing the germs of the papillæ of the *second set of teeth.* * * *

The position of the permanent papillæ, which are at

first situated between the sacs of the deciduous and the gum, gradually recedes behind, falling deeper and deeper, at least, relatively so, as the milk set elongates, until, on the completion of growth in the deciduous, the germs of the permanent set are found in a common alveolus (or socket) at the apices of these cavities, occupying, indeed, almost the position and physiological relations of the original papillæ."

"The first molar of the permanent set is markedly related to the deciduous set, by having a common origin from and in the primitive dental groove; and from sacs, secondary to the capsule of this tooth, spring the reserve cavities of the second and third molars of the second set."

I would only add that there is also formed a delicate membrane covering the enamel of the tooth, called sometimes "Nasmyth's membrane" (from the discoverer), and by Kölliker termed the "cuticle of the enamel," and described by him as being an "exudation secreted from the enamel organ immediately after the ossification of the last enamel cells, which glues together and protects the ends of the prisms of the enamel." Having thus followed the method by which nature forms the teeth, we are ready in the next chapter to study the periods of their eruption.

ERUPTION OF THE TEMPORARY TEETH.

THE temporary teeth having begun to assume their form and dimensions at the fifth month, all of them have begun to calcify at about the seventh month of fœtal life. This hardening process continues, the crowns of the teeth being first completed, afterward the roots. The divisions between the dental sacs also begin to ossify and commence to form the alveoli or sockets, intended as a strong support for the necks and roots.

At that time of the child's life when its growing energies imperatively demand a solid and more strengthening food, the deciduous teeth, which have been forming and calcifying before and since birth, make their appearance.

There are twenty teeth in the temporary set—ten in each jaw. The order and time of their eruption are subject to frequent variation, so that no table can be given which will invariably designate them, but the following may be received as nearly correct in the majority of instances:

4 Central Incisors	from	5 to 7	months	after birth.
4 Lateral Incisors	"	7 to 10	"	"	"
4 First Molars	"	12 to 15	"	"	"
4 Cuspids	"	14 to 20	"	"	"
4 Second Molars	"	18 to 36	"	"	"

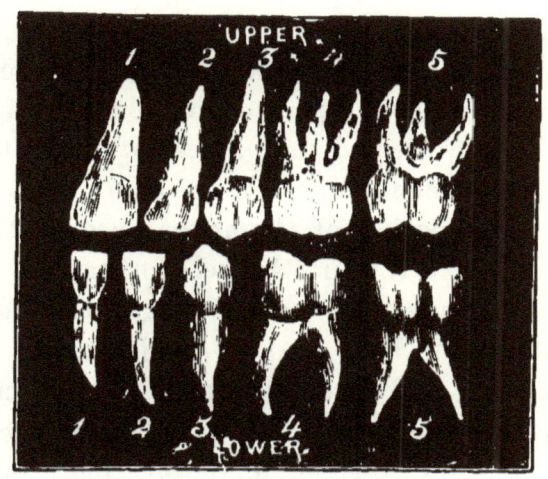

TEMPORARY TEETH OF ONE SIDE.
1. Central Incisors. 2. Lateral Incisors. 3. Cuspids. 4. First Molars. 5. Second Molars.

The cuspids are called also the canine teeth; the upper cuspids are called sometimes the "eye-teeth," and the lower ones the "stomach-teeth." The molars are vulgarly called "jaw-teeth" and grinders. Generally the lower teeth erupt sooner than the corresponding teeth of the upper jaw.

There have been many theories given as to the manner in which nature effects the eruption of the teeth, but it will probably be idle to more than mention them. The longitudinal growth of the pulp for the formation of the root, thus causing pressure toward the surface; the adaptation of the alveolus to the forming root, also causing pressure; and the contraction of the dental sac attached to the gum at one extremity and to the neck of the tooth at the other, thus drawing it through the gum,—are the different supported opinions.

The opening of the gum for the passage of the tooth is caused by the pressure of the sharpest portion of the crowns, and the process of absorption.

As before alluded to, there are many variations in the order and period of the appearance of the temporary teeth, and it would be well for parents to bear the fact in mind. They often begin to erupt very early; some even have been born with teeth. Louis the Fourteenth is a noted example. I have met with some cases in which two teeth have been in the mouth at birth. Then again the temporary teeth occasionally appear very late, being delayed for months, and in some cases on record, for years.

It has been my experience that, in children of anything like healthy constitution, the teeth are more backward where the children are more forward in crawling, walking, etc., and *vice versa*.

THE TROUBLES OF FIRST DENTITION.

THE period from the beginning to the completion of the eruption of the deciduous teeth has long been justly considered as full of mortal danger.

From the bills of mortality collected by Dr. Hufeland, physician to the King of Prussia, in the latter part of the last century, it was estimated that out of every *one thousand* children born, *fifty* died during the time of teething, and *two hundred and seventy-seven* from *convulsions* and *other diseases* during the first two years. Now, considering with good reason that many of those cases of "convulsions and other diseases" were either caused or aggravated by the process of dentition (a fact not so well understood in those days as now), the associated mortality of the period would come near the estimate of more modern times. In France, out of one million of children born, two hundred and fifty thousand, or one-fourth, are said to die before the end of twelve months. In England the statistics tell nearly the same story.

Of course there are many frequently fatal diseases incident to early childhood that are not caused by the irritation of teething, and allowance should be made for them in viewing this immense mortality; but on the other hand this proportion of other causes should not be overrated. Many able men have made too great an allowance, in their argument, that so large a number of infants die *before* the age of six or seven months, the period when dentition generally begins: for it has been shown oftentimes that the teeth at a very early period of their development may produce such irritation and sympathetic derangement of the system, as to terminate fatally in some obscure disease, which *post-mortem* examination has removed the mystery from. Deaths so occurring have been demonstrated to have happened at two or three months after birth. Then, when we consider that *post-mortem* examinations are so seldom permitted in these infantile cases, we are ready to believe that, in many instances, if such examinations should be allowed, we would find that *very many* deaths before the sixth or seventh month could be traced to dentition as the direct or indirect cause.

Writers of our day calculate that of children born, from one-twelfth to one-sixth die during the time of teething. Of those whose vital power enables them to withstand for the time the depressing influence of the period, but whose constitutions are affected thereby to such a degree as to cause them to readily succumb to attacks of disease a few years later, it is impossible to estimate a probable proportion; but it is no doubt a considerable one.

Considering the frail and impressible structure of

the new being, its frequently inherited weaknesses, the improper care taken of it by those intrusted with its nursing, dress, exercise, food and cleanliness; the unhealthy influences of the bad air and contagion of crowded cities, etc., it hardly appears strange that the period of teething should be considered the most critical of life.

To describe in anything like a particular manner all of the diseases which from time to time have been found to arise from the irritation of dentition, would require a special volume; therefore, in this work, I shall confine myself to a simple enumeration of the more frequent troubles associated with the period. And this for the purpose of causing the parent to remember and to be ever watchful for the many enemies that linger around the threshold of his dear child's existence, rather than to offer any suggestions as to the means of baffling them: for this is the duty of the intelligent physician, who should always be summoned at the *slightest* cause of alarm.

Inflammation of the mouth, ulcerative or not, is probably the most readily recognized trouble connected with teething: it may be seen in all stages from that which is simple and localized about an erupting tooth, to the threatening, extending and destructive inflammation, encouraged by constitutional conditions. On account of the mucous membrane extending from the mouth, back over the tongue, palate, tonsils, etc., into the nose, ear and cavity of the eye by certain passages; down the throat into the stomach and intestines; we are prepared to trace back to the irritating teeth certain inflammations, ulcerations and enlargements of parts about the mouth, discharges from the nose, eyes and ears, diseases of the throat, and vomiting, diarrhœa and constipation.

Less obvious to the common observer, but equally obvious to the medically educated man, are other diseases connected with dentition; such as fever, convulsions, skin diseases, hydrocephalus (dropsy of the brain), spurious croup, cough, etc.

Then again there are many diseases, which, though not caused by the constitutional excitement of teething, yet when occurring at the same time, are aggravated, maintained and often rendered fatal by it. Hooping-cough and lung complaints are well-marked examples. All of these and other morbid effects may result from the efforts of a little tooth to burst from its confinement.

Were it not for some violated laws of nature, I doubt not that the irritation of the period of dentition, instead of producing such serious consequences, would serve rather as a healthy stimulation; for it does not seem in accordance with the wisdom of the works of the Almighty, that He should oppress the little, tender infant with a burden so disproportionate to its capacity. As a proof of this we have but to notice the difference of the effects of this process of nature upon the robust children of healthy, compatible parents, surrounded by the invigorating influences of pure air, pure milk, pure water, etc., compared with those of opposite constitution, surrounded by opposite influences. The whole subject demands the close, attentive study of both parent and practitioner. It must be remembered that the nerves supplying the parts in proximity to the teeth are sensitive beyond measure, and moreover that the nervous system of the child is remarkably developed. It should be recollected that the forward pressure of erupting teeth upon sensitive gums, and the backward pressure upon exquisitely sensitive pulps, irritate those nerves. And then it should be remembered that the infant being has no spoken language by which it can express its feelings of discomfort, pain or agony, but that it has another language, no less expressive to those who understand it, the "language of signs and symptoms." How important to comprehend that the variations of the appetite, restlessness, drowsiness, movements of the little hands and feet, knitting of the brows, twitchings of the muscles, movements of the eyes, grinding of the teeth, different kinds of crying, manner of lying, and many other appearances are the forerunners of certain dangerous diseases.

How important to understand that the diarrhœa, or the disagreeable eruption are often connected with the process of teething, and are salutary rather than hurtful, and that to check is to kill.

As I said before, the management of most of the ailments of childhood, during the eruption of the teeth, should be intrusted to the careful physician; but there is one method of treatment about which the dentist is so often consulted and which is so often resorted to by the parent; and which, though so simple and so manifestly beneficial, is yet so often unwarrantably abused and objected to,—that I consider it necessary to say something about it, and will therefore make it the subject of the following chapter.

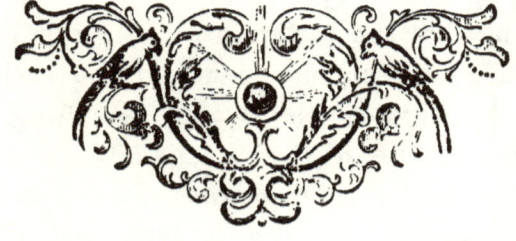

LANCING THE GUMS DURING FIRST DENTITION.

IF any individual should argue that a hot, painful, throbbing boil, tense with irritating matter and producing much systemic excitement, should not be opened; that the operation would be uncalled for and productive of injury instead of benefit, he would not receive much credit for good sense. To the dentist who so often sees the immediate beneficial results of lancing hot, congested gums, the argument that it is an unnecessary operation, productive of irritation and attended with many peculiar dangers, seems just as senseless.

Indeed, when one considers the vast amount of overpowering testimony, accumulated through centuries, in favor of the operation of lancing, as compared with the shallow or imaginary evidence to the contrary, it seems strange that any person should be willing to risk his reputation by arguing in opposition; unless he happens to be of that class hit so well by Goldsmith when he says:

"In arguing too, the parson owned his skill,
For even tho' vanquished, he could argue still."

The operation has been objected to by some on

account of a supposed danger of fatal hemorrhage. Doubtless such accidents have occurred, but how rarely! As many people have bled to death from the extraction of teeth, probably; but so seldom has this occurred that extraction is certainly not considered a dangerous operation. Of ten thousand children in such condition as would indicate the cutting of the gums as a remedial measure, probably one thousand would die if the operation should be refrained from during the whole period of teething; whereas if the gums of the entire ten thousand were lanced *one might* die. No operation should be considered unsafe which exhibits such an infinite number of benefits and such a small proportion of accidents. *Considerable* hemorrhage no doubt frequently occurs, but it yields readily to the proper astringents and appliances.

It has been asserted by others that the enamel of the tooth just before eruption is in a soft state, and is liable to injury from the lance. But this assertion is too absurd to dwell upon, for it is well known to the contrary.

Then, again, some object to incising the gums of the child on account of the pain, fright, struggling and resistance occasioned. Well, I can imagine that a bear in human costume, seizing a young child roughly, forcing open its mouth and tearing a hole in the sensitive gum with an instrument more like a saw than a knife, might produce all of these effects. I know, however, that by the use of great gentleness, the many little playful artifices by which the confidence of the child may be secured, a *very sharp* lance, a dextrous hand and above all *patience*, the operation can be performed with very little trouble, mostly, and often will be gladly submitted to.

A very common objection is that the scar formed by the healing of the incision is tougher and more difficult for the tooth to advance through than the untouched gum. In answer to this, all I have to say is, that in many cases that require lancing, the gum being already on the stretch, the parts open and gradually fall around the advancing tooth; but where a cicatrix *is* formed, it is a fact too well known to be disputed, that scar tissue breaks down much more readily before irritating causes than tissue that has always retained its integrity. The objects aimed at in scarification are to remove the pressure of the advancing tooth, and to relieve the congestion by the abstraction of blood.

In corroboration of the ideas herein advanced as to the usefulness of the operation, I will quote a few passages from excellent authorities. Dr. Chapin A. Harris, in his celebrated work, "The Principles and Practice of Dental Surgery," says: "This simple operation often succeeds after all other attempts to afford relief have failed. We have frequently known children after having suffered the greatest agony for days and weeks, and until they had become reduced to mere skeletons, obtain immediate relief without any other treatment. This at once removes the cause; whereas, other remedies only counteract the effects of the suffering, and can only be considered as palliatives that may assist nature in her struggles with disease, but can not always prevent her from sinking in the contest."

Sir Marshall Hall says: "Better scarify the gums a hundred times unnecessarily than allow the accession of one fit of convulsions from the neglect of this operation. * * * Now, while there is fever or restlessness, or tendency to spasm or convulsion, this local blood-letting should be repeated daily, and, in urgent cases, even twice a day. A skillful person does it in a minute, and in a minute often prevents a serious attack; an attack which may cripple the mind, or the limbs, or even take the life of the little patient, if frequently repeated. There is, in fact, no comparison between the means and the end—the one is so trifling, and the other so momentous."

But, on the other hand, there is no doubt that this useful means of treatment may be abused. Every ailment of early childhood should not be attributed to the irritation of dentition, and the child's mouth continually hacked by indiscriminating persons. Judgment is necessary and certain things should be taken into consideration. The operator should have a knowledge of the time and order of the eruption of the teeth, for although such a knowledge is not an infallible guide, yet it is generally of importance, especially where the local manifestations are not sufficiently marked to indicate the exact spot to which the knife should be applied.

Then where there is supposed to be a hereditary tendency to hemorrhage, great caution should be used, and a course of constitutional treatment would be advisable. It being a well known fact that sometimes erysipelas is developed by small, superficial wounds where there is a predisposition to it, the possibility of its occurrence in some cases should be made the subject of medical advice. If there are no contra-indicating circumstances, and the operation is decided upon, it is easily performed. Much has been written as to the position of operator, assistant and patient and the method of doing it; but a few simple directions are all that are necessary. The operator must have good eyes and a steady hand: the assistant must be strong and reliable. If force is deemed requisite, the child should be placed upon its back across the lap of the assistant, who should secure its hands and feet. The head of the child should be steadied upon the knees of the operator, who should be in the sitting posture. This method of course frightens the child and produces more or less mental distress, but should be adopted without hesitation in case of necessity.

Often, however, the operation can be performed with the child in any posture, by the alternate exhibitions of candy and the lance, or in some other way, and without provoking a cry of alarm or pain. The blade being wrapped nearly to its point, there is no danger of a serious wound being given in case of sudden starting, if ordinary care is used. For each of the six front teeth in either jaw, there should be made a single incision corresponding with the long diameter of the erupting portion of the tooth. For the cuspids a short incision intersecting this at right angles is of advantage. For each of the others (the molars) incisions forming the letter X are required, and these must extend fully to the circumference of the tooth, or even a little beyond. If doubtful as to the exact position of the tooth, a preliminary examination with a sharp needle is useful. The smooth unyielding surface of enamel is readily distinguished from the penetrable bone.

PRESERVATION OF TEMPORARY TEETH.

THE temporary teeth are liable to the same causes of decay as the permanent ones, and equal care should be taken of them. It is really astonishing how little attention is generally paid to them, the prevailing idea being that as they are destined soon to be lost and give place to the second set, it is unnecessary to attempt to preserve them.

This argument as to their loss and replacement is indeed true, but other things of great importance should be taken into consideration. The hopes of the parent are that the anticipated second set shall be placed evenly and beautifully in the dental arches, so that no deformity may exist, that no crowded teeth shall have to be extracted, that no tedious operation for regulating shall be necessary, and that there may be no unusual liability to decay.

Well, then, I give my word for it, the surest way to secure the *disappointment* of all these commendable hopes, is to be negligent in regard to the preservation of the deciduous teeth. It is not the design of nature that the first set shall be lost by the destruction of the *crowns*, but by the destruction of the *roots.* Take care of the crowns and the roots will take care of themselves. It is intended that simultaneously with the advance of the permanent tooth, the absorption of the root of the temporary should occur; so that when the temporary tooth is thus loosened, the permanent one is generally close at hand to occupy its place. Thus no loss of space results, while it would be different if the milk teeth should be extracted months or years too soon; for any one, who has examined at all, has noticed that when a tooth has been lost and nothing has occupied the space, there has been an absorption of the alveolar processes, and a leaning toward each other of the teeth on the sides of the vacancy. Where, then, there is this diminution of space, it is impossible for the second teeth to arrange themselves regularly; there is barely enough room under the most favorable circumstances. Irregularly placed teeth are unusually liable to decay, both from the great difficulty of properly cleaning them, and from the fact that when such portions of enamel touch each other as are not intended to be in antagonism, injury results. How then can the temporary teeth be preserved? The teeth should be cleaned several times daily by the parent when the child is too young to do it, and by either when the child is old enough. Biting into hard candy and holding hard substances in the mouth should be prohibited.

The teeth should be frequently examined by the dentist, and if decay or such imperfections in the enamel as would lead to decay, should be found, the places should be filled. If the child should be too young to undergo the more tedious operation of filling with gold, there are various fillings which are put in in a soft state and subsequently harden, that preserve the teeth sufficiently well, although they more frequently have to be replaced. Besides the advantages, before alluded to, accruing from the preservation of the deciduous teeth, it seems to me that it is not the height of parental kindness to allow children to suffer the agonies of toothache when it can be so easily avoided; nor is it wise to allow their early visits to dental offices to be for the purpose of having their teeth extracted, for often such a lasting unpleasant impression is made that in after years they will suffer their teeth to go to destruction rather than go near the places that are surrounded with such unpleasant associations.

In conclusion, I would state that occasionally there are cases in which the instructions herein given will not hold good, but their occurrence is so seldom that they may be regarded only as exceptions. For instance, sometimes the process of absorption in the roots of the temporary teeth fails to be brought about, and the permanent teeth erupt in front of or behind them; in which case, of course, the solid temporary teeth must be extracted. Then, in certain instances, there is even too much room for the temporary teeth, and a straggling appearance results; when the deformity is considerable, it sometimes becomes a question whether it is not advisable to extract some of the sound temporary teeth, so as to allow the alveolar border to contract, and thus prevent a similar separation in the second teeth. Other anomalies connected with the relationship of teeth to the jaws, and of the jaws to one another, occasionally present themselves, which should be made the subjects of careful study and good advice before determining what course to pursue.

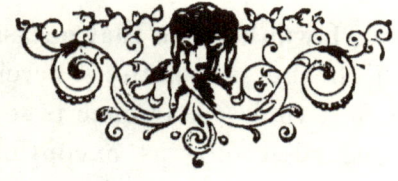

THE PERMANENT TEETH.

THERE are thirty-two teeth in the permanent set, sixteen in each jaw; whereas in the temporary set there were but twenty, ten in each jaw, which completely filled the arches.

In order to make room for the greater number, and larger size of the teeth of the second set, the jaws undergo a process of elongation. By the time that the first permanent molars are ready to erupt (about the sixth year) the jaws have increased in size so as to allow these teeth to take their places immediately behind the temporary teeth. In the portion of the arch, then, in front of these molars are ten temporary teeth; which space is also to be occupied by ten permanent teeth. If all of these second teeth should be larger than the first ones there evidently would not be room for them; but the four incisors and two cuspids are all that are larger—the four bicuspids being smaller than the four molars they take the place of. This, however, will hardly give room enough, and additional space is gained by the crowns of the permanent teeth standing out more in the arch. Many claim that there is also an elongation of the anterior portion of the jaws by the pressure of the advancing teeth. This again has been disputed by just as good authority; but if there is any increase it is certainly a very slight one.

At about the twelfth year the jaws are still further increased in length, so as to permit the second permanent molars to occupy their position just back of the six-year molars. Sometime between the seventeenth and the twenty-first year, generally, the third molars, or "wisdom teeth," erupt in the back part of the arches.

The permanent teeth, beginning to calcify shortly before birth, and continuing to do so for some years, more or less rapidly, and more or less perfectly, according to the state of the general health and the amount of formative material furnished by the food,—erupt about as follows:

First Molars,	from	5	to	7	years after birth.
Central Incisors,	"	6	to	8	" " "
Lateral Incisors,	"	6½	to	9	" " "
First Bicuspids,	"	9	to	10	" " "
Second Bicuspids,	"	9½	to	12	" " "
Cuspids,	"	11	to	12	" " "
Second Molars,	"	12	to	13	" " "
Third Molars,	"	17	to	21	" " "

The incisors are called often in common parlance the "front teeth;" the upper cuspids, canine and "eye" teeth; the lower cuspids, canine and "stomach" teeth; the bicuspids, "small grinders;" the molars, as a class, "large grinders," and the third molars, particularly, "wisdom teeth" or *dentes sapientiæ*. The above table is only an approximation, as many variations occur. Not only are the period and the order frequently irregular, but in some cases the teeth fail to appear at all—the temporary teeth being occasionally retained till advanced life, and sometimes lost.

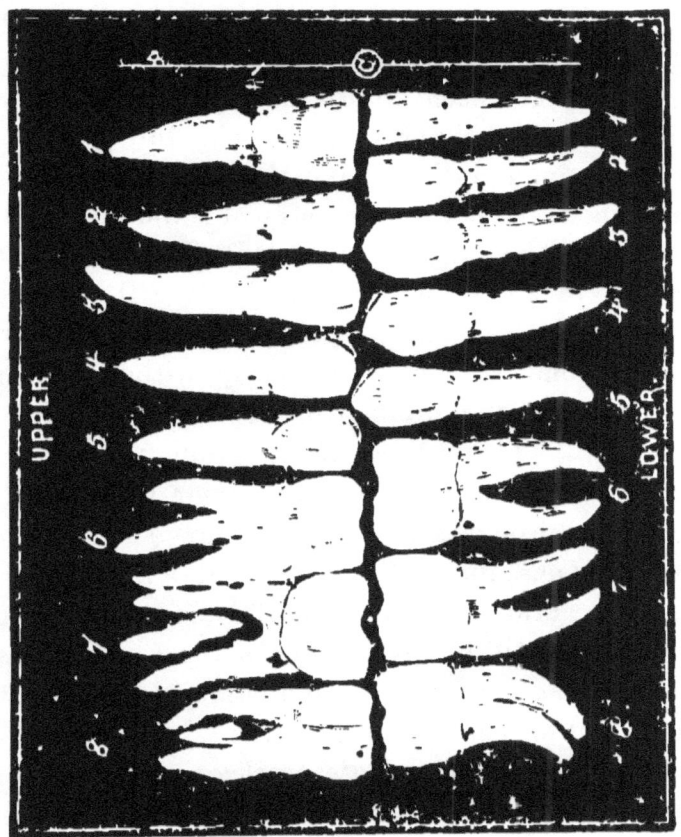

PERMANENT TEETH OF RIGHT SIDE.

C. Center line. 1. Central Incisors. 2. Lateral Incisors. 3. Cuspids. 4. First Bicuspids. 5. Second Bicuspids. 6. First Molars. 7. Second Molars. 8. Third Molars or Wisdom Teeth.

The wisdom teeth occasionally erupt as late as the fortieth or fiftieth year, and sometimes never appear.

Lord Bacon, who lived in Shakespeare's time, seemed to marvel at the peculiarities of "wisdom teeth." In his writings we find: "But divers have backward teeth come forth at twenty, yea some at thirty and forty. *Query* of the manner of the coming of them forth."

Persons have been known in very rare instances to retain certain temporary teeth till thirty or forty years of age, and then have them give way to permanent ones. There is one subject standing mid-way between the first and second dentitions of such importance that I deem it advisable to call particular attention to it. The first permanent molars, four in number, come in most frequently without causing any irritation, and often without the knowledge of the parent. Their time of eruption, as has been seen, is about the sixth year, and their position, back of the second molars of the temporary set. It more often happens than otherwise, that within two or three years after their eruption they decay on account of the bad condition of the fluids of the mouth, caused by the giving away of the temporary teeth and the little attention paid to cleanliness.

In very many cases these teeth are presented for extraction, and it is sometimes impossible to convince the parent that they belong to the second set; the belief being that they are the first teeth because no teeth have been shed to give them place. There is no excuse for such ignorance, and yet it appears that not one parent in a hundred is aware of the truth. I had almost said that not one parent in a thousand knows it, and it is possible that this estimate would be a closer one. It is very essential to save these teeth, and one simple rule will be all sufficient.

Remember that the temporary set consists of twenty teeth, ten in each jaw. Occasionally count them after the fifth year, and when there are twelve teeth in either jaw, *know* that the back ones belong to the second set. Keep them well brushed, and if decay should chance to show itself, have the decayed places substantially filled while the operation can be performed painlessly.

THE TROUBLES OF SECOND DENTITION.

THERE is usually little or no pain or inconvenience attending the eruption of the second set of teeth, as the system by this time has acquired such a degree of vigor and endurance that it is not readily affected as is the feeble constitution of the infant.

Sometimes when the teeth are crowded, there is more or less irritation. And in case that there is not sufficient room for the easy eruption of the wisdom teeth, we have a remarkable exception to this generally easy process of dentition. When this crowded condition exists, and the time comes for nature to endeavor to erupt the tooth, the resistance of some part of the bone or of the adjoining tooth may cause it to take various irregular directions. Violent pain, swelling, throbbing, sore-throat, difficult deglutition, contraction of the muscles, closure of the mouth, periodontitis, alveolar abscess, and general sympathetic excitement are among the minor results; while in some severe cases, lock-jaw, death of the bone and tumors occur.

The treatment that would naturally present itself to the mind would be to extract the offending tooth, if it could be reached, or else the one immediately in advance; but sometimes this is exceedingly difficult of execution, owing to the fact that the jaws are too nearly closed to allow the introduction of an instrument. I call to mind one case in which a young man, afflicted with several of the ailments mentioned above, had been suffering great disturbance off and on for some time; he had been treated for neuralgia and several of the local manifestations, without benefit. Finally, he met some one who had shrewdness enough to suspect that it might be a tooth complication, and he was sent to me with his jaws so nearly closed that I could barely insert the handle of a lance between his teeth. By frequently inserting wedges of gradually increasing sizes, I finally succeeded in opening his mouth sufficiently to extract the second molar of the lower jaw. With the probe I then detected that the wisdom tooth had been growing squarely against the tooth extracted, and, indeed, the form of the crown was somewhat marked on the root it had pressed against.

The dentist should be consulted about the time that the wisdom teeth may be reasonably supposed to be advancing, and preparation made for their eruption, if there evidently should be no room for them. A little timely attention will often prevent a long train of evils.

DESCRIPTION OF THE PERMANENT TEETH.

HAVING now reached the point at which the permanent teeth are supposed to have taken their places in the jaws, some description of them will be in order.

The four incisors and two cuspid, or canine teeth of each jaw are single-rooted teeth. Of these the root of the cuspid is the broadest and longest, and generally has a slight furrow running its length, seeming as if nature had made an attempt at two roots. I have never seen but one cuspid in which there were two well formed roots. The incisors are so called from their broad, *cutting* edges. The cuspid is named from its having a pointed extremity or cusp.

The bicuspid is also generally a single-rooted tooth, but has a deeper groove, which quite frequently divides it into two distinct roots. It is named from the *two* sharp extremities or cusps on its grinding surface. The upper molars have three roots each, two toward the outer surface of the jaw and one toward the inner. There are two roots to each of the lower molars, one presenting behind and the other toward the tooth in front. The wisdom-teeth, or third molars, of each jaw have shorter roots than the other molars, and they generally approach nearer together, frequently forming but one. The roots of these teeth are liable to many deformities on account of their crowded position.

The above description applies to the human teeth in the vast majority of instances, but occasional anomalies occur. I have in my possession a bicuspid with three roots, a wisdom-tooth with four, and a lower molar with three. Upper molars have been seen with four and even five roots.

Concerning the anatomical description of the teeth, that of a simple case, the central incisor for instance, will answer for all; it being remembered that when several roots exist, each one is supplied with blood vessels and nerves, which unite in a common pulp chamber. The hard parts of a tooth are the enamel, the dentine, and the cementum or crusta petrosa. These, as seen in the plate, are so arranged as to leave in the interior of the tooth a pulp cavity containing connective tissue, vessels and nerves.

ENAMEL.—The enamel covers the crown of the tooth, or that portion which is visible upon looking into the mouth. Its substance is arranged in the form of five or six sided prisms; the inner ends face the dentine; the outer are covered and cemented, as it were, by that exceedingly fine but dense membrane, mentioned in the chapter on the Formation of the Teeth. The depth of the enamel is greatest on those

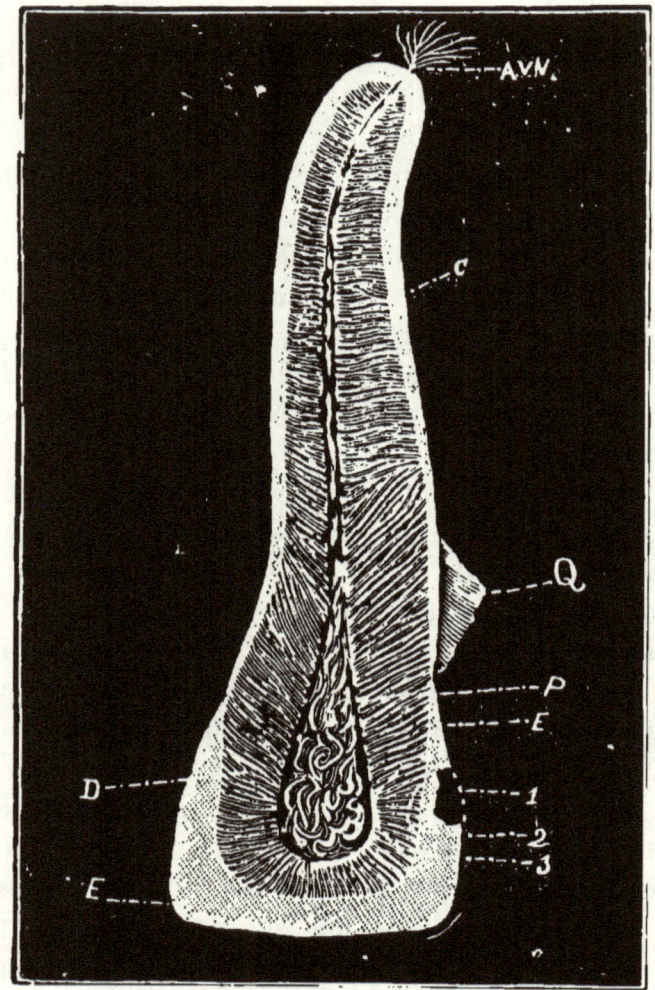

CENTRAL INCISOR DIVIDED AND MAGNIFIED.

E. Enamel. D. Dentine. C. Cementum. P. Pulp. Q. Peridental membrane turned back. A. V. N. Arteries, veins and nerves entering root. 1. Cavity of decay affecting enamel only. 2. Decay reaching sensitive dentine. 3. Decay exposing pulp.

parts exposed to antagonism. It is the hardest of all substances found in living beings, even giving sparks when struck by steel. According to Berzelius, it is made of

Phosphate of lime	85.3
Fluate of lime	3.2
Carbonate of lime	8.0
Phosphate of magnesia	1.5
Soda and muriate of soda	1.0
Animal matter and water	1.0
	100 parts.

DENTINE.—The dentine is never exposed where everything is in a healthy condition, as it is covered in the crown of the tooth by the enamel, and in the root by the cementum. It is not so hard as enamel, but harder than bone or cementum. The greater portion of the tooth is composed of it. Its substance is traversed by innumerable delicate tubes or canals, running from the pulp cavity to the outer surface, conveying fluid and nerve fibrils. It is composed of

Phosphate of lime	62.0
Fluate of lime	2.0
Carbonate of lime	5.5
Phosphate of magnesia	1.0
Soda and muriate of soda	1.5
Gelatin and water	28.0
	100 parts.

It is thus seen that dentine has considerably less earthy matter than enamel, and a greater amount of animal substance; which accounts for the rapid progress of decay when it is exposed. Its nerve fibrils account for its sensitiveness when it is uncovered by caries and irritated by different substances, or by dental manipulations.

CEMENTUM.—This covers the root of the tooth, commencing at the termination of the enamel covering. It is thickest at the end of the root. It is not so dense as the dentine, and approaches true bone in its character: indeed it must to be tolerated by the living parts in contact with it. Were it otherwise it would act as an irritant. Its composition is:

Phosphate of lime and fluoride of calcium.	58.73
Carbonate of lime.	7.22
Phosphate of magnesia.	0.99
Salts.	0.82
Cartilage.	31.31
Fat.	0.93
	10.000

Cementum, having a still greater amount of animal matter than dentine, is considerably more sensitive, as is experienced when the gums are removed by certain causes, leaving it exposed.

PULP.—To this are distributed several small arteries, nerves and veins, which enter at the small opening at the apex of the root. The tubules of the dentine, although too small to allow the entrance of the corpuscles of the blood, yet suck in a certain amount of nutritive fluid. The branches of the pulp nerves divide into the fibrils that enter the tubes.

In addition to the parts of the tooth herein described, we have the peridental membrane which covers the root of the tooth and is attached to the cementum by fibrous prolongations and numbers of vessels. A delicate, structureless membrane has also been detected surrounding the pulp.

IRREGULARITY OF THE TEETH.

A PERFECTLY regular set of teeth is one in which the teeth of both upper and lower jaws are arranged in well formed arches, the upper arch being somewhat larger, permitting the upper teeth to shut a little over or in advance of the lower ones. The cutting and grinding surfaces are about on a line. The cusps and prominences of one set fit into the depressions of the other, so that when the jaws are closed, no important space between them is observable. The incisors and cuspids of the superior jaw are broader than the same teeth of the inferior. This secures an arrangement of the teeth which is of considerable importance in their preservation and in mastication; for the upper central incisors striking against the lower centrals and half of the laterals, and the same relation being observed between the laterals and cuspids,—each of the upper teeth is thereby caused to cover a portion of the corresponding tooth and a part of the next. Thus it will be seen that each tooth, with the exception of the upper third molars and the lower central incisors, is opposed to two in mastication; and that if any tooth is lost, the corresponding one on the other jaw is not entirely useless, as it still antagonizes with a portion of another. This arrangement of the teeth also operates against that effort of nature to expel teeth which have no antagonism. From the regular position of the teeth, above described, there are numerous variations. The irregularity may be so slight as to result in no hindrance to their usefulness, and even be desirable as taking away the suspicion of their being artificial; while, on the other hand, it may be so great as to make the appearance of the person unpleasant or even disgusting. There are various causes for the irregular arrangement of the second teeth, but among the most common are the removal of the temporary teeth too soon, or suffering them to remain too long; hereditary transmission; illness or constitutional disturbance preventing the jaws from growing with a rapidity proportionate to the development of the teeth; suffering the early permanent teeth to be lost; the presence of supernumerary teeth; and the failure to erupt of certain permanent teeth. The teeth of the upper jaw often shut much too far outside of the lower ones, sometimes allowing the front teeth to touch the lower lip, and at other times to come down nearly or quite to the lower gums, completely hiding the lower front teeth when the jaws are closed. Frequently the cutting edges of the upper teeth shut squarely on those of the lower, causing a wearing away and straight edges. In other instances the lower jaw protrudes and the teeth are thrown far in advance of the upper ones, giving a " bull-dog " appearance that is anything but agreeable. Occasionally the back teeth alone antagonize, while there remains a considerable space between the other teeth, which can not be closed by any effort. The incisors, cuspids and bicuspids are frequently seen to have a portion of their number crowded outside of the arch, while others are pushed inside, some of the teeth of the opposite jaw shutting among them in such a way as to lock them in their irregular positions. The same teeth are often turned partially around, lapping over one another, or having their sides presented where the fronts ought to be. In some cases the teeth change places,—the cuspid exchanging positions with the lateral, or the lateral with the central, etc. The failure of certain teeth to erupt, after the loss of the temporary ones, allows their unfilled spaces to be encroached upon by the neighboring teeth, causing a straggling appearance. The same condition often occurs from the loss of teeth by decay or accident, where there is no artificial substitute. Teeth sometimes erupt in the roof of the mouth, and deformed and supernumerary teeth appear in different parts of the arch.

I have confined my remarks to irregularities of the second dentition, for the teeth of the deciduous set are very rarely misplaced. The evil results of these irregularities are many, but I will mention only a few of the most common : imperfect mastication, followed by dyspepsia and other disorders; inability to properly clean the teeth, thus encouraging decay; irritation of the lips, tongue and cheeks; slavering; imperfect speech; inflamed gums; tumors, and disagreeable expressions of countenance. The treatment of the different cases extends all the way from the simple one of letting them alone and trusting to nature, to the most complicated mechanical appliances, assisted by great assiduity on the part of the patient.

Judicious extraction to give room, filing, plates, ligatures, screws, caps, inclined planes, etc., are the means generally employed to correct irregularities; but it will be impossible to lay down any directions which will be applicable to all cases, as there are hardly any two precisely alike.

It can be received as a general truth however, that *any case* of irregularity of the teeth can be either completely corrected, or very materially improved by use of the proper means. The patient should be neither too young nor too old. If too young, the subsequent changes of the growing jaws may operate against permanent benefit; and a lack of the appreciation of the good results would prevent the diligence demanded from the patient in wearing the appliances, keeping them cleaned, etc. If too old, the teeth are so firmly set that it requires a much greater amount of time in which to accomplish a certain result. For anything like a complicated case, I have found from twelve to fifteen years of age to be the best time. Slight irregularities, such as one or two teeth presenting anteriorly or posteriorly, may be undertaken at any time when the child possesses reason and is obedient—the sooner the better.

Probably there is no operation in dentistry that so little attention is paid to, and which the dentist dislikes as much, as correcting the irregularities of the teeth. The objection of the dentist arises from insufficient remuneration, and from the fact that he is often not gratified in the result of his labors on account of the patient failing to co-operate with him, for the patient can not be under the eyes of the dentist at all times, and much attention is necessary in cleanliness, changing ligatures, etc. Then, again, great patience is required in keeping the plate or other appliance constantly in the mouth. Sometimes it has to be worn for months after the deformity is rectified in order to retain the teeth in position until the partially new sockets are well solidified by bone deposit. The dentist being aware of the tediousness of the operation, and the probability that the patient will not perform a proper share of the labor, feels like asking a pretty good fee for taking charge of the case and promising a proper result; whereas the parent, placing too much confidence in the co-operation of the child and himself, and not appreciating the dentist's position, is unwilling to pay so large a price. The proper way to do would be for the dentist to view the case, form his opinion as to how long it would take under the most favorable circumstances to correct the irregularity, and charge so much for that amount of time, without any positive promises as to the result. The charge would thus be exactly proportioned to the amount of labor, and the parent, to whom money is an object, would be stimulated to see that everything should be done that might secure the best results in the limited space of time.

There is another matter connected with the treatment of irregular teeth that demands consideration. Rubber rings are much used around the teeth, and any one who has had any experience, is aware how liable they are to slip under the gums and become hidden. Many a tooth has been lost by a ring slipping from all the teeth but one, and following up the tapering root of that, irritating and loosening it to such a degree that it has been extracted with the cause unsuspected, until the ring has been found far up the root.

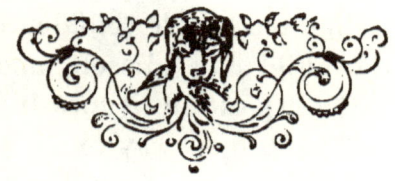

DENTAL CARIES, OR DECAY.

WHEN, at an interesting period in youth, we look admiringly upon a well arranged, clean, sound and beautiful set of teeth, so intimately associated with comeliness of countenance, and contrast their appearance

"Before decay's effacing fingers
Have swept the lines where beauty lingers,"

with that presented a few years later, when from negligence or heedlessness the pearly whiteness has been succeeded by the blackness of decomposition, and the beauty of symmetry has given way to hideous disorder,—we can not but wonder at the unfaithful stewardship of those who so lightly esteem the treasures intrusted to their care.

It is as doubtless the design of nature that the teeth shall endure through life, and perform without material injury all of the labors for which they are created, as it is that the eye, the ear, or any of the members or appendages of the body, shall be able to execute their particular offices until the end of existence. Were the laws relating to the formation and development of the teeth, and their subsequent requirements, fully comprehended and obeyed, they would certainly meet with fewer injuries than any other parts of the body.

The human teeth have doubtless been subject through all time to occasional disease; but it is only of late years that their condition has become such as to cause alarm, and to demand earnest efforts to discover wherein the laws of nature are violated. Let us look at some references to the condition of the teeth in other times. Sir John Sinclair, in his work elsewhere referred to, says: "Former generations seem to have enjoyed a great superiority over the present in regard to the duration of their teeth. A place of interment was lately opened at Scone, near Perth, in Scotland, which had remained untouched for above 200 years, and yet to the astonishment of every one, among a great number of skeletons which were discovered, there was hardly any of them whose teeth were not entire and sound. This is to be ascribed, probably, to a greater simplicity of diet."

John Taylor, a miner at Leadhills, who died in 1770, at 132 years of age, had excellent teeth till within six years of his death. Petrarch Czartan, a Hungarian, who died January 5, 1724, aged 185 years, had some of his teeth remaining. "In Miscellanea Curiosa there is an account of an old man, one hundred and twenty years of age, without the loss of a tooth." Hufeland gives an account of "a lady past seventy years of age, remarkable for the fineness of her teeth, who ascribed their preservation to her

having laid it down as a rule to clean them after
"every meal." These are but a few of the many instances that could be quoted to show that even in days not long past, the teeth were far superior to those of this century; and it is certainly not unreasonable to suppose that those of our times could, by proper attention, be rendered capable of withstanding the wear and tear of an ordinary lifetime. Numerous travelers among various other nations of the globe describe the teeth, even of the now existing generations, as seldom afflicted by disease in those cases where the people live in accordance with the laws of nature, surrounded by healthy influences. In our own country we often hear allusion made to immediate ancestors who retained their teeth to advanced age, and "never knew what the toothache was." In tracing such instances back, we find that the constitution of their bodies was the same as the constitution of their teeth, and that they sprang from robust stock, and remained aloof from the follies of fashionable living. But it is useless to follow these thoughts further; it is our duty to deal with the condition of the teeth as we find it at the present day, and it is a fact that dental caries is generally prevalent, but few sets of teeth escaping its ravages. Teeth have their outward indications of health as well as people, and an experienced observer can tell by certain characteristics their inherent soundness or weakness, and their capability of resisting the various antagonistic influences to which they are liable. The best constructed, most

solid and most durable teeth are of a color just removed from white, with a faint yellowish border near the margin of the gums, gradually shading off into the rest of the crowns, not very large, being of medium width and length; their longitudinal surfaces are perfectly regular on all sides, with no grooves or depressions; their cusps and prominences are not strongly marked; their grinding surfaces have no deep, narrow depressions, and their enamel exhibits no delicate fractures upon the closest examination. Such teeth are seldom attacked with caries, and with ordinary cleanliness and care in their use would rarely have to be taken to the dentist. If all people possessed such teeth, one dentist would be able to perform what a thousand do now, and the other nine hundred and ninety-nine would have to benefit society in some other way.

Teeth of the next best quality are those that exhibit the characteristics of these, with the exception that they have deep depressions or fissures in the grinding surfaces; for though these places are almost certain to decay, they can be substantially filled if taken in time, and the teeth made about as good as those first mentioned. The further the departure from these kinds and the nearer the approach to the pearly white, the chalky, the bluish, or the grayish tinge; to imperfect shape, to length and delicacy of form, to very large or very small size, to pits and grooves on other surfaces than the grinding ones, the more readily are the teeth affected by external influences.

Now, notwithstanding the many different grades of teeth, it has been found by experience that it is a rare thing for teeth to be so poor in quality that they can not be made to last till late in life, by paying proper attention to cleanliness, to the condition of the fluids of the mouth, to the general health, and by visiting the dentist for the purpose of having them examined, and to have them filled at the commencement of decay.

Decay of the teeth is the destruction of their earthy salts from the action of certain corrosive agents. It exhibits different appearances according to the attending circumstances. If the teeth are of solid construction, the decay is darker, and slower in its progress; if soft in texture, the decay is lighter and more rapid in its action. The color varies from nearly black to cream-colored and white. It may attack the teeth at any point, but is much more commonly confined to the grinding surfaces, and the sides or approximal surfaces. I would distinguish decay further by the terms *apparent* and *concealed*; the first applying to that which is readily visible, whether deep or shallow; and the second to that which presents an almost imperceptible opening externally, while inside its ravages extend rapidly, just as a worm eats out the inside of a nut, while only a minute orifice exists in the shell. As will be seen by reference to the plate exhibiting the anatomical structure of the tooth, superficial decay is confined to the enamel covering, or dips but slightly into the dentine. As its depth increases the sensitiveness is heightened on account of the nerve fibrils, and finally the pulp chamber is opened. The sensitiveness and the distance from the pulp depend also upon the position of the decay.

THE CAUSES OF DECAY.

After numerous speculations concerning the manner in which the teeth decay, scientific men have generally come to the conclusion that there is but one essential direct cause, and that is the action of acids. The power of acid to destroy the earthy matter of the teeth may be inferred by reference to the chapter on Phosphate of Lime. The enamel, on account of its extreme compactness, is slowly acted upon; the dentine much more rapidly. If the teeth were always well constructed, with no imperfections in the enamel, it would be safe to say that from acids of such strength as those to which they are exposed, decay would rarely occur, especially as the acids would be so often diluted and washed away by substances taken as drink, and by the continued flow of saliva. But fractures and imperfections of the enamel exist so generally on account of injuries and disease, that the dentine is readily exposed to the action of acids found in the mouth, and from that formed by the decomposition and fermentation of its own organic matter. I probably can not make better use of my time than to quote the interesting and convincing experiments of Dr. A. Westcott, in reference to the effects of acids, etc., on the teeth.

"Both vegetable and mineral acids act readily upon the bone and enamel of the teeth.

"Salts whose acids have a stronger affinity for the lime of the tooth than for the basis with which they are combined, are decomposed, the acids acting upon the teeth."

[A salt is the union of an acid with a substance called a base, each neutralizing the other more or less perfectly, and forming a compound of altogether different properties than those possessed by either constituent. Sometimes the base does not entirely neutralize the acid, in which case the compound is called an acid-salt. Such substances are used frequently as medicines.]

"Vegetable substances have no effect upon the teeth till after fermentation takes place, but all such as are capable of acetic fermentation, act readily after this acid is formed.

"Acetic and citric acids so corroded the enamel in forty-eight hours that much of it was easily removed by the finger nail. Acetic acid, or common vinegar, is not only in common use as a condiment, but is formed in the mouth whenever substances, liable to fermentation, are suffered to remain about the teeth for any considerable length of time."

[Strictly speaking, vinegar is a much diluted solution of acetic acid. Much of the made-up vinegar is very injurious on account of the sulphuric acid contained to increase sourness. The government of England, recognizing this fact, allows the admixture of one-thousandth part only of sulphuric acid.]

"Citric acid, or lemon juice, though less frequently brought into contact with the teeth, acts upon them still more readily.

"Malic acid, or the acid of apples, in its concentrated state, also acts promptly upon the teeth.

"Muriatic, sulphuric and nitric acids, though largely diluted, soon decompose the teeth—these are in common use as tonics."

[In taking any such medicines the teeth should be protected. The method often advised of taking them through a quill is almost useless, as there is always some regurgitation. The proper way is to have a bottle filled with water in which some bicarbonate of soda has been dissolved, and rinse the mouth with some of it before and after taking the medicine. A table-spoonful of soda to a quart of water will be a suitable mixture. Many a set of teeth has been permanently damaged by neglect of such precautions.]

"Sulphuric and nitric ethers have a similar deleterious effect, as also spirits of nitre—these are common diffusible stimulants in sickness.

"Super-tartrate of potash (cream of tartar) destroyed the enamel very readily. This article is frequently used to form an acidulated beverage.

"Raisins so corroded the enamel in twenty-four hours, that its surface presented the appearance and was of the consistency of chalk.

"Sugar had no effect till after acetous acid was formed, but then the effect was the same as from this acid when directly applied."

Besides the acids introduced into the mouth as medicines and condiments, and those formed there by the fermentation of food, the fluids of the mouth are frequently a source, and often there are acid regurgitations from the stomach.

The saliva in its normal state is slightly alkaline, but from certain diseased conditions of the mouth and of the general system, it becomes so acid as to be capable of corroding the teeth with rapidity; as is seen to happen from diseased gums and mucous membrane, disorders of the stomach and bowels, fevers, etc.

It is also subject to other changes which render it liable to putrefy with rapidity and communicate the same tendency to particles of food left in the mouth. This is noticed in bilious, albuminous and puriform saliva, etc.

The thick, tenacious secretion of the mucous follicles of the mouth often produces the same effect.

These facts point out the necessity of having the fluids of the mouth carefully examined in all cases where the teeth appear to disintegrate rapidly and good fillings fail to arrest the decay. Certain tests in the hands of the dentist detect the abnormal conditions of the oral secretions, and often a simple prescription will correct them.

Acids, then, being the direct cause of decay, the various indirect causes may be spoken of as those that injure the texture of the teeth in any way, so as to render them susceptible to corrosion, and those that interfere with the cleaning of them. Besides those that interfere with the healthy formation and development of the teeth, which have been sufficiently considered elsewhere, I will mention the following:

1. Inherited peculiarities. It is well known that certain irregular positions, abnormal shapes, fissures, etc., giving origin to decay, are often transmitted from parent to child.

2. Fractures of the enamel. Cracking nuts, biting threads, falls, blows, the crowding of the teeth in the arch, and many other habits and accidents cause fractures, frequently too minute to be observed by the naked eye, but they nevertheless exist and give entrance to the destructive agent.

3. Roughening and wearing away of the enamel. Picking with metallic tooth-picks, holding pins in the mouth, the pressure of artificial plates and clasps, the use of powders containing too much grit, all produce a scratched or worn condition of the enamel.

4. Swollen gums. Old roots of teeth and the sharp edges of large cavities of decay frequently irritate the gums, causing them to rise up on the sides of sound teeth, thus forming a place for the lodgment of food and acids; they also vitiate the

fluids of the mouth generally by their contaminating influence. Accumulations of tartar often act in the same way. Swollen and inflamed gums moreover commonly prevent the use of the brush on account of pain and bleeding. Connected with this subject, it may be mentioned that the wisdom teeth, on account of deficiency of room, are often only partially erupted, the gum forming a lid over a portion of the crown.

5. Badly performed dental operations. Sometimes in filled teeth, the metal instead of just filling the cavity and being continuous with its exterior margin, overlaps and forms a crevice in which injurious agents secrete themselves. At other times the cavity is not full enough or the metal is not well consolidated. Occasionally, through indiscreet use of the mallet, the enamel at the margin of the filling is fractured and subsequently disintegrates. After the use of the file in separating, finishing fillings, etc., the scratched surfaces are often not sufficiently polished. The same remark will apply to the condition of the enamel sometimes observed after the removal of tartar by scaling instruments.

This enumeration includes the most common causes of decay, but before closing I will mention two others that have been the occasion of considerable discussion of late years—galvanic action and infusoria and fungi. That a small galvanic battery may sometimes be formed in the mouth from the presence of two different metals, one of them being acted upon by the oral fluids, no one can deny. As a proof of this is given the familiar experiment of Sulzer, a century old, of placing a silver coin above the tongue and a piece of zinc beneath it; a little electric shock and peculiar taste occurring when the metals are pressed into contact. But that such galvanic action generally exists, and that it causes the wholesale destruction of the teeth that the extremists claim, I have not the courage to assert; especially when I consider the fact that such claims could be so well refuted by many whose teeth have remained in a comparatively good condition for a quarter of a century, notwithstanding the juxtaposition of different kinds of metallic fillings. I have no doubt, however, that in many cases slow, and, sometimes, rapid injury results when the position of the fillings, the acidity of the fluids and the quality of the tooth substance combine in the most favorable manner for galvanic action and decomposition.

Concerning the infusoria and fungi there is no doubt of what the microscope has proven to exist in abundance in the human mouth. In fact, cavities of decay have been spoken of as minute aquaria, teeming with animal and vegetable parasites. Whether they cause decay or not has never been definitely settled by disputants. My opinion is that they do exert some influence, and I am led to believe this from consideration of the fact that they possess the power of destroying organic matter, as is seen in the occasional destruction of gold-fish and the tails of reptiles to which they attach themselves.

THE PREVENTION AND CURE OF CARIES.

THE great method of prevention is to keep the teeth clean. To secure proper cleanliness, pleasant taste and purity of breath, the teeth *ought* to be cleansed *five times* a day; once after each meal, once before retiring and once during the morning ablutions. In the morning the brush and good powder should be used and the mouth rinsed. After each meal all particles of food should be picked from between the teeth, and then the brush and clean water will be sufficient. At night the brush and water will answer, occasionally using a little good Castile soap and then rinsing the mouth. The best toothpick is one made from a quill, but after using it should not be kept in the mouth the balance of the day, till it is mashed into a ragged brush. The tooth-brush should be applied so as to reach *every accessible* surface of the teeth and so as to brush the food from *between* them; therefore it should be used backward and forward and from side to side on the grinding surfaces to clean out all the depressions; and upward and downward in the divisions between the teeth, inside and outside. Once or twice a week, or oftener, a silk thread armed with powder should be drawn between all of the teeth. So well do people generally appreciate the necessity of keeping the teeth clean, that about one in ten thousand takes such care of them. One of a thousand, probably, goes through the form of cleaning them three times a day. A greater number clean them once a day, and that in the morning, allowing the food from three meals to accumulate, putrefy and ferment all day and all night till the next morning again. But the great majority of people don't clean them at all and—glory in it often. Many that do pretend to brush the teeth, rattle the brush along the row, just as a boy rattles his stick along the palings; this does about as much harm as good, packing the particles of food and decomposing mucus nicely away between the teeth, and leaving untouched the grinding surfaces. It would be just as sensible to attempt to paint a fence by rubbing the brush across the pickets instead of up and down. Many who have been careless with their teeth will doubtless think that to follow these directions will be an arduous duty, but the attention here advised will not require in the aggregate more than ten minutes of each day; and after a little while it will assume the form of a habit and will be naturally added to the ordinary routine of daily duties. The dentist should be seen occasionally, that he may remove deposits of tartar, see that the gums and fluids of the mouth are in a healthy condition, and that there is sufficient room between the teeth to allow them to be cleaned; also that he may examine the condition of the teeth in places that the patient can not see.

When from any cause, decay does occur, the means of cure are filing, burring and filling, operations that will be spoken of in full hereafter.

Finally, if people would fully realize the truth of that aphorism given to us by Shakespeare:

"A little fire is quickly trodden out,
Which, being suffered, rivers can not quench,"

and would pay more frequent visits to the dentist, we would seldom see those cases of aggravated decay, agonizing toothache, offensive breath, early loss of the teeth, etc., that have become so common. The majority of people *will* wait until pain drives them in desperation to the dentist to have teeth extracted that could have been saved without peradventure and without pain, if they had been filled in the early stages of decay.

It is sufficiently near the truth to lay it down as a rule that a small spot of decay, unattended to, is as sure to end in the destruction of the tooth, as a small fire is sure to end in the destruction of the building.

A decayed tooth *never* repairs itself, and to save it the dentist *must* be patronized. One great popular mistake is that the teeth are not decayed as long as they give no pain; whereas pain comes from the advanced stages of decay. It is a common thing for a patient to go into a dental office confidently asserting that there is *only one* decayed tooth in the mouth, when examination will detect a dozen. It is *utterly impossible* for patients to examine properly their own teeth; to do it requires delicate mirrors and fine instruments that the uninstructed can not use, and an angle of vision that can not be employed.

Expense, which is such an object to many, and

which is so much increased by delay, ought to be a strong appeal for the necessity of early attention.

Ten dollars will often do at one period what will require a hundred dollars a year later.

"An ounce of prevention is worth a pound of cure;" "Great ends from small beginnings grow;" "A stitch in time saves nine;" and a whole volley of proverbs and maxims could be hurled at the unbelieving and indifferent. "*Time* is money," and an hour or two in the early stages of decay is only consumed, instead of days at a later period. *Pain* is the dread of mortals, and early operations are *painless* where later ones are *painful*. *Beauty* and *comfort* are preserved at one period; whereas they are lost at another. Then besides, it should be remembered that bad teeth are often attributed to a lack of cleanliness, and

"Cleanliness is indeed next to godliness."

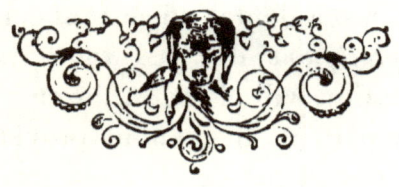

FILLING, OR PLUGGING.

AFTER the removal of the decomposed matter from a cavity of decay, the operation of introducing metal, or some other substance, for the purpose of arresting the further progress of the disease, is called filling. Considering the countless instances in which good fillings have preserved the teeth in excellent condition ever since they were put in many years before, it is really astonishing that so many persons still live in ignorance of the usefulness of the operation. Many there are who through ignorance or prejudice suffer their teeth to go, one by one, suffering meantime the agonizing tortures of toothache, most offensive breath, vitiated saliva, impaired digestion, impure blood, and numerous other evils, and are at last left toothless and with general derangement of the system. In some cases the prejudice has arisen from their own, or their parents' experience in early days, when the operation was not so well understood, and good dentists were scarce; making no allowance for the great improvements that have taken place in materials and in the qualifications of the operators. Many through parsimony or poverty have had their teeth poorly filled with cheap materials, and by cheap dentists, and are unwilling to believe that fine fillings, inserted by skillful hands, will give better satisfaction. Others again have allowed their teeth to proceed to exposure of the nerve or ulceration of the root, before having them filled, and because they did not turn out well, condemn all filling as useless. It would be just as sensible to call in a physician in the last stages of some fever, and because the patient does not recover, refuse to believe in the healing power of medicine; or to let a house burn nearly to the ground, and because the engines can not save the property at that late hour, declare them incapable of ever accomplishing good. Some won't have their teeth touched because their first experience gave them so much pain,—not realizing that small cavities are generally not painful, or that means have been discovered to allay sensitiveness. And a great number, after having had their teeth filled once, have since had no regard to cleanliness, suffering their teeth to decay around the plugs and elsewhere, and blame the dentist for what is attributable to their own negligence.

Filling the teeth with the right material, in the right manner, and at the right time, will almost invariably save them, if the patient co-operates with the dentist by doing his part of the work afterward. In any case, it is more certain than any remedial operation that can be performed upon any other portion of the body. A person may be treated for any disease and restored to perfect health, but there is no certainty that he will not be attacked by another the next day or the next week; whereas good fillings at the proper time are almost sure to preserve the teeth from *any* disease for a number of years. Every one should know what is essential in a good filling, that he may be able to judge whether the work is well or poorly executed, and know whether to blame the dentist or not, should the operation prove unsuccessful. All decomposed and soft substance should be removed from the cavity. The cavity should be shaped so as to be but slightly wider internally than at the entrance, no matter how much cutting away has to be done, for it is impossible to introduce the instruments so as to thoroughly condense a filling in a cavity that has a large area of decay inside, while the external margin describes a very much smaller circumference. Besides, the thin plate of enamel which, under such circumstances, would be left over the filling, would be very liable to subsequent fracture. Teeth very often decay in the manner spoken of, for the hard enamel is slowly acted upon, while the softer dentine is eaten away rapidly, and many such teeth are improperly filled by timid dentists, who dare not cut away the enamel for fear of being accused of unnecessarily enlarging the cavity in order to secure a greater fee.

The work ought to be done well, even if the future patronage of a suspicious patient should be lost.

The margins of the enamel should be smooth and

firm, so as not to crumble under the necessary pressure. After syringing all the débris from the cavity and making it completely dry, the filling material should be pressed into every inequality, and the entire filling thoroughly condensed, so as to perfectly exclude the atmosphere, fluids and particles of food. The filling should then be dressed down so that its edges may be exactly even with the surface of the enamel, being neither too low, too high, nor overlapping. It should then be well smoothed and polished.

If the filling is on the masticating surfaces it must not be felt when the jaws are closed tightly together; if on the approximal surfaces, enough space must be left between the teeth to allow cleaning. When the work is finished the patient must do his part by keeping the filling clean, otherwise it will be liable to have decay renewed around it.

A finely polished steel blade, if left in a damp cellar, will become covered with and damaged by rust; it may be taken out and by proper labor have its brilliancy restored, but it would be foolish to place it right back where it would be subject to the same damaging influences.

The dentist should be called upon every few months that he may examine his fillings, and see whether the fluids of the mouth, the care of the patient, and all the surrounding conditions and circumstances are favorable to their preservation; for every honorable practitioner takes a pride in his operations, and is anxious that his work shall be perfectly done. But how can he take an interest in his labors for a patient who remains away for a long time, taking no care of his teeth, and finally comes back growling about his fillings coming out, and wanting him to do them over again *for nothing,* when he has given his dentist no chance for observing the quality of his work? Many people keep away from the dentist because they are afraid that he will find something to do, never considering that they ought to be glad if he does; for time, pain and expense are saved by early operations. Dentists do not charge for examinations and consultations, although there is no reason why they should not be remunerated for time occupied in professional advice, as well as physicians or lawyers.

Various materials are used in filling teeth, each of which possesses some advantages that the others do not, and neither of them answering *every* requirement necessary to constitute a *perfect* filling in all respects; perfect adaptation, natural color, hardness, lack of shrinkage, non-conduction of heat and cold, uninjuriousness to the teeth, mouth or general system, and unchangeableness in mastication, or from exposure to anything with which it may come in contact. I will mention these different materials separately, and give my opinions as to the relative merits and advisability of each, untrammeled by any personal preference, and regardless of the prejudices of others.

GOLD.

The preparation of gold for the use of the dentist has become a distinct branch of business. It comes to us in the form of leaves of various degrees of thickness, being adhesive or non-adhesive; also, in soft spongy masses called on account of slight differences in appearance and manner of preparation, crystalline or sponge, plastic and shred gold, all of which are very adhesive. Adhesiveness is the name given to that quality of gold, by which one portion, by pressure, becomes so incorporated with another as to make a mass almost as solid as coin; but sometimes this property is objectionable, as in deep and narrow and irregular cavities difficult of access, for the gold becomes consolidated before it is pressed into all the inequalities. Adhesive gold foil and sponge gold are peculiarly applicable for contour fillings, or those in which a lost portion of the tooth has to be built up to its original shape; but it is much more tedious to use them than the soft gold, and great care has to be used to keep them from getting wet, as the least moisture ruins their adhesive properties.

The fillings made of them, when proper'y done, are the perfection of skill and beauty, as any shape can be imitated and a most lustrous finish can be given. Non-adhesive gold answers well in many cases, especially in the masticating surfaces of the bicuspids and molars where there is no building up to do, and it is much easier of introduction; but it is not susceptible of so fine a finish, and is more apt to crumble out when once started from any cause, as by picking, and by fracture of the enamel at the edge of the filling.

Gold is unquestionably the best material that has ever been employed for filling the teeth, and may always be considered the most appropriate in cavities sufficiently easy of access where the pulp is not too nearly exposed, and where the walls are firm enough to allow the pressure necessary for perfect consolidation. It can be adapted to every minute portion of the cavity, resists perfectly the force of mastication, exerts no evil influence upon the teeth or any other part, and remains entirely unchanged from any agency with which it is liable to come in contact. This is more than can be said of any other material.

Pure gold put in the teeth to-day, will be pure gold in the grave a thousand years hence. Its color in front teeth is very objectionable to some whose tastes are such that they prefer to have tooth-color fillings many times renewed, or even to have artificial teeth, rather than to show the burnished gold every time they move their lips. Its power of conducting sensations of heat and cold to a sensitive pulp is sometimes a serious disadvantage, the continued irritation occasionally producing in it inflammation, loss of vitality and suppuration; but proper medication, and the interposition of some non-conducting substance between the filling and the location of sensitiveness, will generally prevent such occurrences.

In filling very large cavities requiring a great deal of pressure and malleting, there is no doubt that occasionally the peridentium is thereby injuriously excited, especially in people of great susceptibility to irritating influences. Another objection that sometimes exists to the use of gold is, where the walls of the cavity are so thin and brittle as to make it questionable whether or not they are able to withstand the required pressure, for it will not do to compromise matters and insert an imperfect, half-consolidated filling, just for the name of having gold in it. Finally, the expense of well executed gold fillings is an impassable barrier to many who fully appreciate their teeth, and would have their work done in the best manner if they could afford it. The question, what to do in such cases, constantly presents itself to the mind of the dentist. I can not but condemn the practice of those operators who, clinging obstinately to their theory of "gold or nothing," drive away such patients and compel them to go to the cheap charlatan for cheap fillings, poorly inserted. Other fillings than gold, well put in by a skillful dentist, and well taken care of by the patient, will often save the teeth for a considerable time, perhaps until the days of prosperity.

Of course, it is difficult sometimes for the dentist to know whether the patient is poor or penurious, but he should have the benefit of the doubt, and whether he is unable or unwilling to pay the price of gold, he should have the dentist's best services in something else; especially as the patient is the one who has to suffer in case of any misrepresentation.

TIN FOIL.

This is probably the next best metal for *preserving* the teeth in anything like simple cavities with strong walls. Its color is much less agreeable than that of gold, even when first put in; but in many months it is soon chemically affected, turns black and disintegrates. Its softness is such that it is readily conformed to the shape of a cavity and makes, therefore, at first a good filling, and very often lasts as well as gold. It is better than gold as far as its conduction of thermal changes is concerned. Its lack of adhesiveness renders it unserviceable for any but the simpler kinds of cavities.

FUSIBLE ALLOYS.

Tin, cadmium, lead and bismuth melted together in certain proportions form a compound looking much like lead, and is fusible at a very low degree of heat. For instance, when placed on paper and held over over a flame it melts without the paper being scorched. The cavity being kept perfectly dry, is filled by piece being added to piece by means of warm instruments. Unless through mismanagement, the heat is not sufficient to cause any unpleasant sensation. It preserves its color well, can be built up to any shape, and where a good foundation is secured it makes a fair filling. As it is not much used, I have never felt sufficient interest to examine particularly, but there is doubtless some little contraction of the filling on cooling, which makes it liable to have decay started around it. It is used genera'lly as one of the dernier resorts in the worst cases of carious teeth. It possesses some advantages over amalgam, in that it is not suspected of evil effects, can be entirely dressed and polished at one sitting, and is easily removed in case after trouble renders it necessary. Such fillings sometimes last many years.

GUTTA PERCHA.

GUTTA PERCHA alone, and in combination with feldspar, quicklime, etc., is frequently used for temporary fillings, and as a non-conductor beneath metal filings. It is applied with warm instruments in the manner described for fusible alloy. Hill's stopping and White's preparations are those most commonly used. Such fillings are soft and unirritating, and are excellent for temporary purposes, and sometimes, indeed, last for several years.

OXY-CHLORIDE OF ZINC PREPARATIONS.

OS-ARTIFICIEL, osteo-dentine, bone-filling, white-filling, osteo-plastic, cement-plombe, Guillois' cement, etc., are some of the names applied to a certain class of compounds consisting essentially of oxide of zinc combined with silex, borax and titanium and other coloring matters, made into a paste with chloride of zinc just before using; and which hardens in a few minutes.

The number of these compounds indicates the great longing for a perfect material for filling teeth, or one which combines the natural color of these preparations with the many good properties of gold. These plastic materials are superior to gold in some respects. They match very nearly the different shades of the teeth, so as not to be distinguishable at a little distance. They adhere to the walls of the cavity so firmly, that its shape makes but little difference. They allay the sensitiveness of the teeth by the pain-obtunding action of the chloride of zinc, which is often used by itself for that purpose; for this reason os-artificiel is often happily used in those cases, especially among females, where the sensitiveness of the teeth is excessive from sympathetic association, and where the existing condition makes it unadvisable to go through a long and tedious operation of gold filling. What it lacks is the durability of gold, for it is gradually, within a variable time, removed by the fluids of the mouth. It is much used as a covering for exposed pulps, the permanent filling being placed over it. It is this application of it that has caused such a great amount of discussion in our conventions and associations for several years; one party arguing that it invariably devitalizes the pulp, while the other declares it to be harmless. As for myself, I believe that it will nearly always destroy it if applied in immediate proximity to it, sometimes when the pulp is separated from the filling by but a small amount of tooth substance, and hardly ever when the pulp is well protected. Excellent fillings are made in certain kinds of cavities by filling the greater portion of them with oxy-chloride of zinc and finishing with gold, being in all respects as good as when made entirely of gold. Numerous cases are reported of oxy-chloride of zinc fillings being perfect at the end of from five to ten years. Doubtless there is difference in the quality of different lots of the material, but I think the main cause of its early failure in the hands of many dentists, is in not keeping it perfectly dry for several days by covering the filling with some impervious coating. I consider it a valuable acquisition to the dental profession, and more advisable than any other filling in front teeth much disfigured by decay, and where doubts exist as to the permanency of gold.

AMALGAM.

As connected with dentistry, this name is applied to a paste made of silver and tin filings and mercury. It has for years been the subject of more discussion than any other material used by the profession. To represent fairly the opinions of its enemies and advocates would consume a volume. Saying nothing of its injurious local and systemic effects, it is certainly the greatest curse that ever has been visited upon the dental profession. Being easily mixed, readily plastered in some fashion into a cavity and setting in spite of moisture, it has long been used wherever the laziness or incompetency of the dentist, the poverty or illiberality of the patient, the pressure of time or the difficulty or impossibility of using gold has caused a decision against the latter metal. It possesses one superiority over gold or anything else, and that is hardness, being harder often than the consciences of those who unreservedly use it. Many of the effects of mercury manifested so distinctly in the coppery taste, swelling, tenderness, and ulceration of the gums and tongue, profuse flow of saliva, loosening of the teeth, gangrene, sloughing of the soft parts, death of the bone, etc.; or seen in mercurial palsy, characterized by convulsive agitation, difficult speech, mastication, locomotion and vision, debility, blackening and decay of the teeth, etc. (which effects so frequently have arisen from the administration of the medicinal preparations of mercury and from exposure to its fumes), have so often been traced to the presence of large quantities of amalgam in the mouth, that it is folly to deny its power for evil. It is a worthless argument that the quantity of mercury absorbed from fillings is too small and extended through too long a time to produce its peculiar effects; for searchers after the truth are well aware that this gradual accumulation of mercury in the system is what produces the serious effects so often noticed in the cases of button and other gilders, looking-glass makers and other workmen.

There is frequently a much greater amount of mercury put into the mouth in the shape of fillings, than often is required to produce injurious effects when administered in medicines or used in ointments for skin diseases. Some persons are peculiarly susceptible to the effects of mercury, not being able to bear small doses of it, while others can take much larger quantities with impunity. It is generally conceded that more cases of root troubles, as abscess, periodontitis, etc., occur in teeth filled with amalgam than in those filled with any other material; but the fact that a much larger proportion of badly decayed teeth are filled with amalgam than with other substances, interferes with the value of this testimony. Galvanic action from the presence of different metals in the mouth, has been alluded to in another article. With amalgam fillings and the fluids of the mouth, we have the requisites of a miniature battery.

The power of voltaic electricity to decompose compound substances is exemplified in the experiment of the decomposition of water; the current being sent through this liquid, hydrogen is given off at one pole and oxygen at the other.

Of course the power of the mouth battery is very feeble in comparison with that used for chemical experiments, but when the associated conditions are favorable, it is no less certain. It is not difficult to imagine how acids may be formed from the union of elements set free by this process of decomposition. Hydrogen and oxygen being liberated from combination in the water of the fluids, the hydrogen combining with the chlorine from chloride of sodium in the saliva, forms hydrochloric acid. Nitrogen, from decomposing food uniting with the oxygen from the water, forms nitric acid. Besides the formation of acids destructive to tooth substance, other effects may occur. The chlorine of the chloride of sodium of the saliva and of the chloride of potassium of the mucus, uniting with the tin and mercury of the amalgam, forms chlorides of these metals, which, being soluble, are washed out, thus accounting for the porosity often observed in old amalgam fillings. This porous condition, and the shrinkage from the walls of the cavity that occurs during the hardening of the amalgam, open the way for further decay.

One of the great objections to amalgam is its unseemly appearance when it becomes very much discolored, as happens in the majority of mouths. This discoloration is attributable not only to the action of agents formed within the mouth, but also to certain kinds of food. Mustard, eggs and some kinds of game discolor the amalgam just as they discolor silver spoons and forks, owing to the action of the sulphur contained in them. I have thus endeavored to point out the worst effects that may happen from the use of amalgam, especially from a common article; the best qualities are made from chemically pure materials and contain less mercury than the others. But the most violent opposers of amalgam have no doubt allowed their zeal to carry them to too great an extreme. To say that the use of amalgam, even in considerable quantities, is *always* productive of great injury and fails to preserve the teeth, is asserting too much. While writing upon the present subject, I have had occasion to examine the mouth of a gentleman whose teeth are in a most excellent state of preservation, and yet he has more than a dozen good sized amalgam fillings that were inserted as many years ago by some dentist in whom he had great confidence, and who imposed upon his credulity by telling him that amalgam was much better than gold. Considering that the amalgams of that time were so much inferior to the best of the present day; that they are now hardly discolored at all; that he has had gold fillings put in his mouth since, which ought to increase the galvanic action; and that his health has always been remarkably good, and his teeth have never given him any trouble; it is certainly a well marked instance to prove that amalgam fillings sometimes do good service. It is no uncommon thing to meet persons with a less number of such fillings, which have preserved their teeth for nearly double the time. Upon the whole, however, it is my firm conviction, considering the idiosyncrasies of different individuals and the effects that often do follow the use of amalgam, that it should never be used except in moderate quantities, as a last resort, or as temporary fillings; and then preferably for persons that will take good care to keep their teeth clean and their mouths in good condition, occasionally visiting their dentists that they may examine the condition of the fillings and remove them if need be. The amalgam paste should be thoroughly washed by working it in a mortar with soda, chloride of zinc or alcohol until all impurities are removed; the surplus mercury should be well squeezed out and then the same care should be taken in shaping the cavity, putting in the filling and finishing when hard, as with gold. A few words in reference to the removal of old amalgam fillings. Their hardness is proverbial, and it is distressing to hear of the tedious operations that have often been submitted to in having them drilled and cut, if not blasted from the cavities, by dentists that did not know that by scratching the filling so as to obtain a clean surface, and then adding some new soft amalgam paste, the old plug will soon be so much softened that it can be readily cut out.

SENSITIVE DENTINE.

The varying degrees of sensitiveness exhibited during operations upon the teeth of different individuals, have long been a matter of surprise. One patient will take his seat in the dental chair and have his teeth probed, drilled, burred, and hammered for hours, retaining his composure with stoical indifference, and, possibly, going to sleep; while another whose teeth are not nearly so badly decayed, will wince at the slightest touch, and writhe with agony at the necessary application of power, pronouncing the pain unbearable and refusing to submit to further manipulations. It is not worth while to enter into any speculations as to the causes of the peculiar susceptibility to impressions existing in certain people; it is no more to be wondered at that the teeth should possess such peculiarities, than it is that many other parts of the body may, in one person, endure almost pleasurably, sensations which would be very disagreeable or insupportable to another. The nerves which supply the teeth (fifth pair) are the most sensitive of any in the human body, and it has been previously shown that the terminal fibrils of these nerves are the ones that ramify through the substance of the dentine.

When such excessive sensibility occurs, no matter how provoking it is to the dentist to have the patient twist and start at every touch, it is useless to get angry, or to attribute it to affectation, lack of self-discipline or childishness; the loss of *patience* often results in the loss of *patients*. Whether the person can not or will not stand it, it is the duty of the dentist to endeavor to relieve the hyper-sensitiveness, and remove that dread of dental operations that exists in the minds of some people to such an extent, that they can not be induced to go near a dentist except for that last resort—extraction, and even that must be done under the influence of an anæsthetic.

If the patient can possibly summon the resolution to allow the decayed matter to be cut away by a few vigorous strokes, I believe it to be, generally, the best way; but if not, medication should be resorted to. Apropos of this subject, I would mention how dangerous is that habit, often indulged in by patients, of suddenly and forcibly dashing their hands against that of the operator, as an indication of unwillingness to submit to further operations. There is danger of making an unsightly wound, or of putting out an eye. If they can not or will not submit to the pain, the manly or the womanly way to do, would be to slowly and firmly take the hand of the dentist, interrupt his work and decidedly refuse to allow him to proceed. Different substances have been used as local applications to sensitive dentine. Sometimes it happens that one fails to answer the purpose in some cases, when it does admirably in others.

The patient should not give up at the first trial, but experiment with all of the recommended applications; for it rarely happens that some one of them does not succeed. The most of these act by destroying the vitality of the outer portions of the animal matter of the dentine, and forming a more or less insoluble compound with it, which remains as a pellicle protecting the parts below. Creasote and carbolic acid (nearly the same preparations) are much used and are excellent. The odor and taste are objectionable, but the idea that they cause decay of the teeth is erroneous. They only affect the animal matter, and in reality preserve it, as the creasote of smoke preserves meat. Chloride of zinc is another. It is in general use, and very reliable. The dangers of inflammation and destruction of the vitality of the pulp have been spoken of before. Nitrate of silver is often applied. Sometimes the discoloration of the cavity, which it blackens upon the same principle that it does the skin, is an objection. Tannic acid is often a good remedy, as is terchloride of gold. Arsenic is the surest agent, but many refrain from using it on account of the danger of its causing the death of the pulp, even when left in but a little time; not at once, but subsequently from the absorption of what finds its way into the tubules. If applied in very minute quantities, well secured in the cavity, and left in but an hour or two, when the nerve is not too nearly exposed, being afterward well syringed out and an antidote applied, I believe that injuries of any kind would happen so seldom that they need not be taken into consideration. But on account of the careless manner in which it is often applied, and the neglect of patients to have it removed at the proper time, other means should be tried first. Cobalt, which owes its action to the arsenic contained in it, is considered safer. Hydrate of chloral, perfectly harmless and unirritating, has been tried with considerable success. Instruments heated from warm to red-hot have been found very efficacious, but this method has never been regarded very favorably by the patient.

Sub-cutaneous injections and internal administration of small quantities of morphia, have been found to produce the best results, on account of their controlling influence over the nervous system. The remedies mentioned in this chapter should be applied only by the dentist, as great care is required in the use of most of them. The condition of the saliva should be looked into, as this often has much to do with the abnormal sensitiveness of exposed dentine.

CAPPING EXPOSED NERVES.

WHAT is called the *nerve* of a tooth, in common parlance, is in reality the *pulp*, consisting, as has been previously seen, of several minute arterial, venous and nerve branches; but for the sake of being better understood, I will adopt the erroneous term for a caption, rather than insist on correct nomenclature. Destroying the nerve, bleeding the nerve, etc., are errors of the same kind. Not many years ago the majority of the members of the profession believed and taught that when decay had once encroached upon the pulp, it was impossible to preserve it alive, and that, before filling the tooth, the exposed pulp had to be devitalized. I am sorry to admit that many believe, or at least *teach* the same thing nowadays; whether they lack the patience, the knowledge, or the skill requisite for saving the pulps alive, I will not decide. To secure success, a knowledge of the anatomical structure of the teeth, their physiology, and the treatment applicable to their diseased conditions, is certainly required; and often, moreover, great patience and skillful, precise, and delicate manipulations are demanded.

It is certainly no exaggeration to assert that the majority of teeth that have had their pulp cavities recently exposed by decay, or have been opened into while doing the necessary amount of excavating preparatory to filling, and have not settled down into cases of chronic toothache, may be preserved with undiminished vitality. Further than this, a fair proportion of the most unfavorable cases can be restored by proper medication to a condition healthy enough to justify permanent filling. It will probably be unnecessary to urge the importance of saving the pulp.

The tooth is nourished in two ways; partly by the sustenance it receives from the membrane covering the root, but mostly from that derived from the vessels circulating in the interior. If the supply from the latter is cut off, the outer membrane is stimulated to increased action, and will often maintain the vitality of the tooth for some time, but frequently it fails; the tooth is then necrosed, or dead, and becomes a source of irritation. A living tooth is just as much better than a dying one, as a living tree is better than a dying tree; the latter, after girdling, fails to bear foliage or fruit, although it may continue to rear aloft its lifeless and decaying branches for some time.

The principle involved in preserving the life of the pulp, is the protection of its sensitive structure, by placing over it some non-conducting, unirritating substance to prevent the access of air, food, heat, cold, or any of the exciting influences to which it is exposed,—and then filling the cavity in a substantial manner. The pulp then often co-operates in this design of protection, by going to work in the privacy of its little chamber, now protected from the intrusion of impertinent visitors, and repairing the breach in the dentine by the deposition of new bony matter, just as it deposited it during the period of the formation of the teeth.

The pulp being free from pain and hemorrhage, and the surrounding associated parts in a healthy condition, there are various methods of operation that promise success. After touching the exposed point with a little creasote, a lead, gutta percha, or gold cap, having a concavity that prevents its touching, may be placed over it. Then the cavity may be filled with either a permanent or temporary filling; the latter is generally preferred, as it is less irritating by not requiring as much time or labor, and if there is no trouble after a reasonable length of time, it may be removed to give place to the permanent filling. A properly shaped piece of quill, or a drop of collodion from which the ether evaporates instantly, leaving a pellicle, are excellent non-conducting substances to interpose.

A small piece of letter paper saturated with creasote, over which is placed a little asbestos, is another.

In case of threatened inflammation after the operation, often a little judicious treatment will counteract such tendency. Lancing the gum around the tooth to relieve the fullness of the vessels; lying with the head a little higher than usual at night, and taking a warm foot-bath, to promote the flow of blood from the head; holding a piece of pencil rubber, or some other substance between the jaws at a distance from the seat of trouble, so as to prevent the irritation of antagonizing teeth; are remedial measures that should not be neglected. Besides these, it is often very beneficial to have an application made by the dentist of the tincture of iodine and aconite. A saline cathartic, as epsom salts, is often invaluable.

An appreciation of the value of a living tooth should prompt a person to endeavor by every effort to retain it in that condition; but if after reasonable trial the hope has to be abandoned, then the pulp may be devitalized and removed, and the tooth filled with a fair prospect of preservation for a sufficient length of time to fully justify the operation.

Another method sometimes adopted to preserve the pulp from inflammation and suppuration after filling, is to drill a small hole at the margin of the gum into the root as far as the canal, care being taken not to wound the lining membrane of the pulp; but the success attending the operation is not sufficient to recommend it as a remedial measure of much value.

ROOT FILLING.

It sometimes happens that the pulp is so exquisitely sensitive that it will not tolerate the presence of the most unirritating caps or non-conductors; at other times when presented to the dentist, it is already dead, having lost its vitality spontaneously, from the irritation of a previous filling, from frequent medication to cure toothache, or from some other cause. In such cases shall the tooth be extracted or shall an attempt be made to save it? A few years ago extraction would have been advised in nearly every instance. Some can be found who advise the same thing in these days. But the experience of the best operators, throughout the world now, teaches that the percentage of success attending rightly performed root-filling operations is so great, that it is good practice to attempt to save almost every tooth with a dead pulp that presents itself. If alveolar abscess has resulted and continued for a long time, the case is much more complicated, but even then it is often astonishing what nature will do when assisted by proper local and general treatment.

It is very much a matter of the appreciation of the natural teeth by the patient, and the manner in which the work is done by the dentist. The vast majority of failures is doubtless attributable to the imperfect manner in which the operation is performed, the patient frequently not being willing to consume the time or put himself to the inconvenience of making a number of visits to the dentist for the necessary dental treatment; or if willing to do these he is often not willing to give the dentist sufficient compensation. The following is a description of the manner in which the work is ordinarily done. The patient through neglect suffers a tooth to decay until the pulp is exposed and the tooth aches; he then goes to his dentist to have the tooth extracted, but is informed by him that there is a probability of saving it. This the patient is desirous of doing, if it does not take much time from his business and does not cost much. So an arsenical preparation is applied and he comes back in a day or two to have it removed and the tooth filled. The pain is entirely gone and everything looks favorably; perhaps the nerve and vessels are partially removed from the canal, perhaps not; the cavity is then filled either perfectly or imperfectly, and the patient goes on his way pleased with the result. In the majority of such cases, at some subsequent period, varying from a few days to several months, root trouble manifests itself, either from not having the tooth and membranes restored to a healthy condition, or from allowing more or less of the dead pulp to remain in the canal to putrefy and irritate the investing membrane of the root. Even at this period a removal of the filling and *proper* treatment would probably succeed, but the patient is not willing to risk it again and the tooth is sacrificed to the forceps. Now let us take a case in which both operator and patient do their whole duty to secure the best prospects of success; the one possessing the requisite skill, patience and appliances, the other willing to take the necessary time, and able and willing to make a reasonable remuneration. Let the suppositional case be that of an upper molar which has decayed in such a manner as to expose the orifice of only one of the root canals. The paste of arsenious acid and morphia, which is the agent generally used, placed in the cavity will destroy the vitality of the pulp in all of the canals; but when the time comes for removing the paste and the dead pulp, the three canals can not be reached from the original cavity; it must be much enlarged, or a new cavity drilled into the grinding surface. The canals, always small, are sometimes so minute that the finest instrument can not be made to enter them; but they must be enlarged and the contents entirely removed to the end of the roots. Medicines must then be applied until any irritation caused by the tedious labor is allayed. Frequently, applications are required to correct the putrefaction of small portions of decomposing matter that are unavoidably left in the curves of the most tortuous canals.

After everything is brought to a healthy condition, the three roots, one by one, must be thoroughly filled with gold, or some other material, and afterward the cavity in the crown. It is not always advisable to do the filling at one long sitting, but to divide it into several sittings. It is often a better plan to put temporary fillings in both roots and crown for several months, and then if no trouble arises, to remove them for permanent fillings. Many dentists prefer to make the permanent fillings in the roots of cotton and creasote, claiming that they preserve the tooth just as well, while they possess the great advantage of being readily removed in case of after trouble, thus giving another trial for the preservation of the tooth. The great difficulty and sometimes the impossibility of removing well condensed gold fillings from such narrow canals, can be readily imagined. The above remarks apply of course as well to teeth, the pulps of which are dead at the time they are presented before the dentist, only they generally require a longer course of preparatory treatment; especially if alveolar abscess exists. Seeing then the much greater amount of skill, time and labor required in such a complicated case, compared with the filling of an ordinary cavity, and that the dentist ought to be better paid for an operation perfect in all its details than one that is not,—the question arises whether or not the dentist is justifiable in putting in the filling in the crown, and slighting the root, in those cases where the patient is unable or unwilling to pay for the best services. Dental statistics seem to show that he is, for some teeth so filled never give any trouble, and when the others do there is yet a chance for filling them properly; or if it is decided upon to extract them, it is no more than would have been done in the first place; besides, the fillings strengthen the teeth and render them less liable to fracture under the pressure of the forceps. Before leaving this subject, I would say a few words as to the propriety of filling roots, the crowns of which have been broken off or have decayed entirely away. If left in their ragged or decayed condition, they are a constant source of evil to the fluids of the mouth, to the soft parts and to the adjoining teeth. If the roots are in front and are solid enough, they should be made the supports of pivot teeth. If the other teeth are crowded and irregular, or if artificial teeth are advisable, they should be extracted. Otherwise, much good often results from smoothing and polishing them and filling the canals; they can be thus kept perfectly clean and maintain the position of the other teeth.

MALLET FILLING.

AMONG the many recent improvements in dentistry, which render the competent operator able and even anxious to undertake complicated cases of gold fillings, which a few years ago the best dentists would have given up as impossible, the mallet occupies a prominent place. There are two kinds of mallets, the hand and the automatic. The first is shaped somewhat like an ordinary hammer, and is used by an assistant to strike against an instrument held by the operator, the force of the blow being transmitted to the filling, and condensing it better and more expeditiously than hand pressure. They are constructed of either wood, lead, ivory, or other material, but which is best has not yet been decided to the satisfaction of all parties, although the members of different dental conventions have spent several years in trying to mallet into each other's heads the superiority of certain kinds of mallets. The automatic mallet consists of an instrument with a hollow handle, in which is placed machinery for striking against a movable point inserted in the end of the instrument. Certain screws and slides graduate the force of the blow. This instrument is used by one hand of the operator, and requires no assistant. It possesses some advantages over the hand-mallet; it can be used in some positions where the other can not; there is no liability to accident from a mis-stroke; and it is more comfortable to the patient, as there is perfect regularity in the strokes, and there is no worry of mind as to whether the next blow is going to be harder or lighter. But in the majority of cases it does not do its work as well as the hand-mallet, on account of the quivering nature of the blow; it is very useful, however, in certain places. The hand-mallet gives that sure and solid blow, when properly used, that is calculated to perfectly condense a filling; but it must be wielded by an experienced hand; an accidental sidelong blow on the end of the plugger may throw the point to one side or the other, and break off or crack a portion of the tooth, as may a blow before the operator is quite ready. The employment of mere children to use the mallet has always appeared to me reprehensible. No dentist can perfectly signify to another person before each blow just what kind he wishes, whether hard or light, quick or slow, lingering or rebounding; therefore, the malleter should see the cavity and have had some experience in filling teeth. The mallet, although such a valuable adjunct, is nevertheless liable to abuses. It may be used so indiscreetly as to fracture the walls of the cavity; it may occasionally by its jarring irritate the membranes connected with the tooth; but the principal injury arising from its use is that which often occurs in the last part of condensing, where care is not taken to avoid minute fractures of the enamel at the edge of the filling. As before mentioned, in speaking of the causes of decay, the fractures may be too small to be observable to the eye, but exist to a sufficient extent to admit destructive agents, which in the course of time undermine the fillings.

It is true that this same injury may arise from violent and misdirected hand pressure, but it is not nearly so liable to occur.

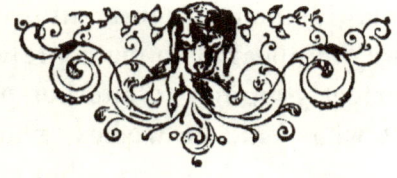

THE FILE.

PROBABLY there is no operation in dentistry that encounters so much opposition as the use of the file.

Patients generally consent to its use very reluctantly, while many have their aversion so strongly set, that no reasoning will cause them to yield.

There is no doubt that a great amount of mischief may result if the operation is performed in a bungling and imperfect manner, but that is true of filling, extracting, or any other operation in dentistry. On the other hand, however, there is no better preventive or curative means within reach of the dentist, than the file used in the proper cases, and in the proper manner. The prevailing opinion is that when a portion of the enamel is removed, decay is certain to occur; this is controverted by too many facts. Many barbarous nations file their front teeth to sharp points for the purpose of better tearing their food to pieces, and also, as they think, of adding to their beauty; yet these very people are remarkable for the soundness of their teeth. The enamel is thick enough to bear considerable cutting without exposing the underlying dentine, but even if the latter should be uncovered there is not nearly so much danger of decay as is generally believed, if the surface is kept clean. Every dentist of much experience has seen numerous instances in which all of the teeth separated by the file have remained entirely unaffected by caries, while all of the corresponding teeth in the same mouth that were not so separated, have decayed in a few years, although they were perfectly sound at the time of the filing of the others. The sides of the teeth would probably not decay once, where now they decay a thousand times, if they were separated early by the file, and the surfaces frequently cleansed. When the teeth are crowded too closely together, they not only wear one another in the slight movement that all teeth have in mastication, but they prevent the passage of anything between them for the purpose of removing the destructive agents which work unmolested on the affected enamel. A very small space is all that is required—just sufficient to pass a thread through with comfort. The practice of filing the teeth heroically away, seemingly to show defiance to the unfounded prejudices of the opponents of filing, is censurable, both because it is unnecessary, and because of the disfigurement. The separation should not be made clear through to the gum, the teeth being allowed to touch there; otherwise they would come together again. The work should be done with fine files, and the enamel afterward made as smooth as possible with powders, burnisher, etc. Rubber, wooden wedges, etc., are frequently used to separate the teeth for the purpose of filling them, but the file should be used also to prevent subsequent touching. Superficial decay can often be removed by the file, and it should always be done where disfigurement of the tooth will not follow. The burr-drill is but a modification of the file, being an instrument with a small ball-end, which is file-cut; it is useful in removing incipient decay, where the resulting concavity would not be so deep as to be difficult to clean. Natural teeth that are too long for correct articulation with artificial ones, and elongated teeth that have no antagonists, have to be shortened by files; roots are also dressed down by them for the insertion of pivot teeth. Excessive local and general sensitiveness can generally be controlled by medicines.

SEPARATING.

When decay occurs in the approximal surfaces of teeth which are crowded very close together, it is necessary to separate them before the cavities can be cleaned out and filled properly. There are different methods of procuring this necessary separation.

Some prefer to quickly force the teeth apart with wooden wedges; others, to do it slowly by inserting from day to day, wedges, or pieces of rubber or cotton of gradually increasing sizes. Many consider the use of the file the best method.

Each has among its advocates some of the best operators of the day. Patients also have their preferences and prejudices. It is not my intention to contest these different views, but I can not refrain from giving my opinion as to the best means of separating the teeth, based upon my own experience in practice, and upon examination into the results of the methods adopted by others.

Each has its objectionable features, but I believe that the judicious use of the file, generally gives better satisfaction to both dentist and patient, than either slow or quick wedging. There is no doubt that wedging very often produces inflammation of the peridental membrane, sometimes inflammation and death of the pulp, and occasionally permanent displacement of the teeth. These results never follow the right employment of the file. Teeth that have decayed on account of their crowded condition, coming back to their original position after the removal of the wedge, are just as liable again to decay around the fillings; unless the latter are left convex to prevent the teeth from coming together, which often occasions the disagreeable sensation of something crowded between the teeth and constant picking to remove it. If the file is not used as it should be, far greater injury arises than from the employment of wedges, and it is doubtless from such faulty operations that most of the prejudice against this useful instrument has arisen.

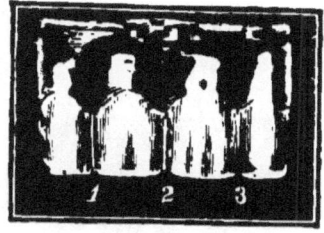

The accompanying figure represents how the teeth should be separated by the file and how they should not be. If the cut is made clear through below the margin of the gum as at No. 1, the teeth will come together, and further decay will almost infallibly result. The separation should be made as at No. 2, where a slight shoulder prevents the teeth from coming in complete contact, although the points will probably touch. No. 3 represents a still better form where the decay has not extended too near the points of the teeth. Often slight wedging in conjunction is advisable. It is surprising to see the inconsistency sometimes exhibited by the champions of wedging when they denounce the use of the file in all cases, and yet separate the teeth by wedges, and then file the filling down even with the enamel, roughening the tooth just as much as if they had filed it in the first place, and yet not securing sufficient space to prevent further decay. When approximal cavities exist in the front teeth with no anterior disfigurement, many operators prefer to cut away a large V shaped space at the back of the teeth and fill them at that point. This is doubtless the best method, as it causes no division in front and forms a space behind that is almost self-cleansing. The following figure represents the rear view.

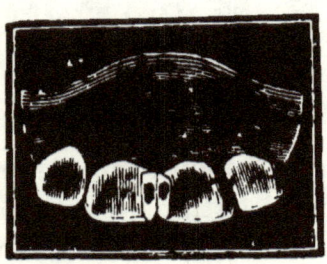

COFFER DAM RUBBER.

VARIOUS instruments and appliances for facilitating operations, and adding to the comfort of patients, have been invented for the use of dentists. It seems useless to mention them, as every operator should be supposed to have all improvements that are calculated to make his work better in quality and easier to himself and patients. But there is one improvement, comparatively recent, that deserves particular attention, both because it is not universally used by dentists, and because in many cases it is so very essential to the comfort of the patient. This is the rubber-dam, introduced by Dr. S. C. Barnum. The difficulty of controlling the flow of saliva used to constitute one of the greatest objections against tedious and complicated fillings. Stuffing the mouth with napkins, and holding down the tongue and closing the salivary ducts with compressors, have always been regarded as very disagreeable. Even these failed to check the oozing of moisture from the gums about the necks of the teeth, and many fillings have been ruined by becoming thus wet before completion. In the majority of cases, by the use of the rubber-dam, inconvenience and unsuccessful operations may be avoided.

It is but right that the patient should know of and demand the employment of any appliance that does so much toward the removal of the dread of dental operations. The first of the accompanying figures shows a sheet of the rubber with holes punched in it for allowing the teeth to slip through, and the second gives a representation of the teeth with rubber-dam applied.

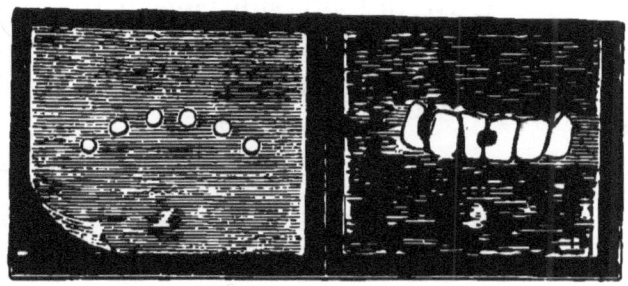

It will be seen that the contraction of the rubber around each tooth effectually precludes the access of moisture into the cavities of decay, while at the same time the patient is not bothered with napkins and has the liberty of moving the jaws and swallowing.

BLEACHING THE TEETH.

TEETH which have become discolored from the chemical decomposition of amalgam fillings, from the infiltration of dead pulp substance, or from the stains of certain topical applications, can generally be restored to their original color by the use of bleaching agents.

These operate by uniting with some element of the coloring compound, thus decomposing it.

Solution of chloride of soda and diluted nitric acid are the agents generally employed. Oxalic acid is peculiarly applicable where the discoloration is attributable to the salts of iron. Cyanide of potassium has also been used for bleaching. All of these substances require great care in their use, and as some of them are very destructive to tooth substance if their effects are not counteracted, and also injurious to surrounding parts, they should never be applied except by a dentist.

SALIVARY CALCULUS, OR TARTAR.

CALCULUS, derived from the word calx, a stone, is the name applied to solid concretions appearing in any part of the body. Tartar is the name given to hard deposits in casks containing fermented wines. Thus is seen the origin of the terms used in dentistry to designate those earthy depositions around and on the teeth. The source of tartar, and the cause of its being deposited, have been the subjects of much inquiry, and have never yet been so satisfactorily settled as to hush discussion. The theory supported by the large majority is that it comes from the true salivary secretions, and in proof of this we have the fact that it is most abundantly deposited upon the outer surfaces of the upper molars and upon the inner surfaces of the lower front teeth, close to which the ducts of the parotid, and of the submaxillary and sublingual glands, respectively, enter the cavity of the mouth. Some claim that its deposition is due to the fact that the saliva being alkaline, and containing the phosphate and carbonate of lime, these are precipitated when the saliva comes in contact with the acid mucous secretion.

Others assert that in certain conditions of the system there is a superabundance of earthy matters in the saliva, which mechanically settle upon any surface to which they can attach themselves. Dr. Garretson believes that "when the salivary secretions are sluggish, the inorganic material, not being held in solution until fairly ejected into the mouth, becomes deposited about the roughened and inviting surfaces of immediately neighboring teeth." This theory seems unreasonable to me, both because I have observed that often, in the worst cases, the salivary flow is considerably augmented, and because if it were remarkably sluggish, and deposition resulted therefrom, stoppage of the ducts would be very liable to occur, which, comparatively speaking, seldom happens. Other authorities abandon altogether the idea that salivary calculus proceeds from the saliva, and claim that it owes its origin to the secretion of the mucous membrane, or from small glands whose particular office it is to secrete the substance. Dr. Schrott, a celebrated German dentist and microscopist, ascribes the origin of tartar to the presence of the infusoriæ of the mouth; and after speaking of the locations where the deposit is most abundant, he says: "These places are also the true places of meeting for the infusoriæ; here they remain the longest time, obtain their highest age, die, and their living remnants interlace with epithelial cells, parasites, remains of food, slime, and secretion of saliva, and form, in this manner, the tartar of the teeth."

But leaving these probable and improbable theories, let us come to the subject of tartar as it exists, its effects and its treatment. In the mouths of different individuals, it differs much in regard to quantity, effects, rapidity of accumulation and appearance. On one extreme, the deposition may be so slight as to be scarcely noticeable; on the other, it may be so great as to completely hide several of the teeth, flying off in large masses when disturbed by instruments. It varies in color, being black, several shades of brown and yellow, and whitish. That which is black in color is the hardest and most tenacious; the lighter it is in color the softer it is. The white tartar, and a certain green stain found generally on the outer face of the upper front teeth, are the most injurious to the teeth themselves, corroding the enamel and causing speedy decay. The other varieties cause little or no injury to the enamel, but are very injurious in many other respects.

Salivary calculus, even when not directly affecting the teeth, is very injurious to the gums, sockets, breath, secretions of the mouth, the general health, etc. The first deposit irritates the gums; they inflame, suppurate and withdraw; here they would stop and heal if it were not for the continued addition of tartar which causes the gums to recede more and more. This deposition also encroaches upon the vessels which supply the membrane affording vitality to the alveolar processes and the roots of the teeth; the devitalized processes are gradually absorbed, and finally when they and the gums are both gone, the teeth are past saving, and are ready to drop out. So intolerably offensive does the breath become from some kinds of porous tartar which give lodgment to decomposing mucus and food, that it is almost insufferable by any one but the happy owner. The fluids of the mouth becoming vitiated are taken into the stomach, which rebels at such a condiment; the blood becomes full of impurities, the system suffers, and often the best efforts of the physician fail while the cause exists. Dr. Harris, in his work on dental surgery, further enumerates the effects of salivary calculus as follows: "Tumors and spongy excrescences of the gums of various kinds; necrosis and exfoliation of the alveolar processes, and of portions of the maxillary bones; hemorrhage of the gums; loss of appetite, derangement of the whole digestive apparatus; foul breath; catarrh, cough, diarrhœa; diseases of various kinds in the maxillary antra and nose; pain in the ear; headache; melancholy, etc." Add to these, closure of the salivary ducts, periodontitis, alveolar abscess, and various sympathetic pains; think a little—and then resolve to keep the teeth clean. There is one great means of present cure, and that is the operation of scaling performed by the dentist. The common inquiry put to the dentist is: "Does it not injure the teeth to scrape them?" Of course it does—a *little;* so it does to clean the rust from a knife, but it is certainly far better to do it than to allow the rust to remain till there is nothing left to clean. Much depends also upon the manner in which the scraping is done; just as a man *might* be shaved by having hair, skin and all scraped off, while a more gentle tonsor might be kind enough to leave the skin.

Some of the deposits have so little attachment to the enamel that a slight touch with the scaler detaches the mass in a single piece, leaving the enamel smooth underneath; other kinds so corrode and become incorporated with the teeth, that they lose a part of their substance in cleaning. Every particle of tartar must be removed, and if the enamel is at all scratched it must be polished with powders and burnished. If the gums have become inflamed and cover the lower margins of the deposit, several sittings may be required before the gums have sufficiently healed to allow all of it to be visible. After the tartar is removed, and between the sittings, a healing wash should be used. There is one great means to prevent the reaccumulation, and that is to keep the teeth clean. There is no disguising the fact that excessive deposits of tartar proceed from negligence in this respect; it is at first creamy in consistence, but afterward hardens if not removed. Explicit directions as to the manner of cleaning the teeth are given elsewhere. Slight accumulations may occur in certain locations in spite of care; the dentist should then be visited.

ODONTALGIA, OR TOOTHACHE.

THE term toothache is generally used to denote any kind of pain which arises from a morbid condition of the teeth, or of the membranes connected with them.

The causes of pain connected with the teeth are so various, and the remedial measures' for each so different, that scientific exactness calls for some systematic classification; consequently, professional men have distinct names for the different diseased conditions which produce tooth-pain. The peculiarities of nature are nowhere noticeable to a greater extent than they are in the different effects produced by irritation of the parts associated with the teeth. In some cases, almost imperceptible causes produce unendurable agony, banishing sleep and appetite, occasioning various constitutional disturbances, and often, doubtless, so debilitating the system that the entrance of disease is rendered easy. In other instances, conditions may exist which would be considered capable of producing the most serious effects, and yet only slight discomfort, or none at all arises. The pain may proceed from only one tooth, or from several at the same time; or it may flit from one to the other. It may last for a long time almost without intermission, prompting the sufferer to resort to all kinds of positions and all kinds of applications, in the vain effort to obtain relief; or it may come periodically and go away of itself, or yield when a certain position of the body is assumed or when a certain local application is made. It seems that the vocabulary of adjectives has been exhausted in searching for names to express the different kinds of toothache; digging, shooting, boring, cutting, throbbing, jumping, thumping, tearing, gnawing and pulling, are some of them. Odontalgia arises mainly from sensitive dentine, irritation of the pulp by external agents, pulp nodules, periodontitis, alveolar abscess, decomposition in the pulp cavity, fungous pulp, fungous gum, exostosis, exposed cementum, necrosis, and sympathy.

Sensitive dentine has already been treated of at some length in a previous article connected with the operation of filling the teeth. It is only necessary to add that the dentine may become exposed in other ways than by decay or by the excavation of a cavity for filling; thus fractures may occur in which a piece of the enamel is chipped off, or it may be exposed by denudation and abrasion, affections which will be mentioned hereafter. Too much filing may also expose the dentine. Though often not sensitive when laid bare, yet at other times it is exceedingly so, and the contact of hot and cold substances, sweet and sour things, the atmosphere, etc., produce considerable pain.

IRRITATION OF THE PULP BY EXTERNAL AGENTS.

In the anatomical description that has been given of the pulp, it has been seen that it is composed principally of delicate arteries, veins and nerves. Various causes may occasion an increase of the blood which is distributed to it, just as a greater flow may be brought to the skin or other parts by irritating causes. The walls of the pulp cavity being solid and unyielding, expansion is prevented and pressure is made upon the nerves, which produces pain. The amount of this pain depends upon the size of the opening at the apex of the root and the calibre of the vessels which enter, the extent to which the circulation of the blood is augmented, the nervous susceptibility of the patient, etc. The pulp may be irritated in many ways. Particles of food, hot and cold fluids, draughts of air, etc., may come in contact with it in cavities of decay. Even if protected from the direct contact of these by a considerable amount of decayed matter, the decomposed dentine may irritate by actual impingement and by conduction, or it may allow the ingress of acids. Metallic fillings may convey impressions of heat and cold to it, or they may be inserted with so much force as to bulge in or break thin walls of protective dentine. The occasional action of the chloride of zinc in os-artificial fillings, has been already alluded to. The progress of the spontaneous or mechanical wearing away of the teeth, beyond the point of exposure of sensitive dentine, may produce inflammation of the pulp. Blows and falls, and fractures in attempts to extract teeth, often expose the pulp. Exposure to cold and wet may, by contracting the superficial vessels, produce an increased circulation in it.

The same means that are used to combat determination, congestion and inflammation in other parts of the body, are equally applicable to the treatment of the dental pulp in the same conditions. Anything that diminishes the quantity of blood in its vessels, will often be immediately beneficial: thus the warm foot-bath draws blood to the opposite part of the body; counter-irritation by blisters, etc., answer the same purpose; or the blood may be directly drawn by frequent lancing of the gums, pricking the pulp, application of leeches, etc. Cathartic medicines, by producing liquid discharges from the bowels, reduce also the amount of blood in the system. Applications of cold by constringing the vessels, force out the surplus of blood when the diseased condition has not progressed so far as to interfere with the free movement of the fluid. The position of the body has much to do with the circulation, as has often been experienced by those who have had to pace the floor at night, or sleep in the sitting posture, positions which favor the reduction of the circulation in the vessels of the head. Concerning the local applications to cavities of decay encroaching upon the pulp, the list is almost endless. From the many remedies may be selected spirits of camphor, turpentine, laudanum, ether, chloroform, tincture of aconite root, oil of cloves, creasote, and acetate of morphia. Dr. Harris gives in his work a good prescription:

"℞. Sulphuric ether, ... 1 fluid ounce.
 Powdered camphor, ... 2 drachms.
 Powdered alum, ... 2 drachms.
 Sulphate of morphia, . . . 2 grains.

"The alum should be very finely powdered, and all the ingredients well mixed before use. After removing all foreign matter and carefully drying the cavity of the tooth, a small bit of cotton or lint dipped in the above mixture may be applied, and renewed several times a day if necessary." The same directions are appropriate for the application of the other remedies. Another useful prescription, that may be put up for family use, is this:

℞. Oil of cloves, ... 1 fluid drachm.
 Sweet spirits of nitre, . . . 1 fluid drachm.
 Acetate of morphia, ... 10 grains.

The mere removal of the irritating decayed matter, and stopping the cavity with wax or cotton, will often relieve the toothache; or where the irritation is caused by the acid contents of the cavity, the application of a little bicarbonate of soda, or some other alkali to neutralize it, is frequently all that is necessary. The application of anything but the simplest remedies should rarely be attempted by the patient, for to secure good results, the cavity ought to be well dried, and the tongue and cheeks kept out of the way; the medicine should then be protected from the entrance of saliva by some impervious substance. The tincture of aconite root is very poisonous, and a few drops taken into the stomach may produce alarming results.

It is distressing to see the injury that patients sometimes do themselves by the careless use of creasote, badly burning the lips, cheeks and tongue. If such accident should occur, sweet oil should be immediately applied. A drop or less is all that is needed for any tooth, and it should be well secured in the cavity; the shape of this is often such that it is impossible for the patient to properly apply the medicine.

The remedies mentioned generally give only temporary relief, and it is no uncommon thing for a patient, before going to the dentist, to suffer off and on for weeks, trying meanwhile every conceivable remedy, passing many sleepless nights, and at last desperately calling for extraction. He is then often in such a frame of mind that he will listen to no promises of saving the tooth; his spite has accumulated to such a degree that it can only be pacified by having the blood of the offending member. The right course to pursue would be to go to the dentist at first, and have the pulp capped and the tooth filled. The simplicity of the treatment depends much upon the length of time that has elapsed since the commencement of trouble, whether or not the peridentium is affected, and upon the condition of the general system; but it is safe to say that a great number of pulps can be saved alive even after exposure, while in the great majority of cases, extraction is certainly rendered unnecessary by the ability of the dentist to devitalize the pulps and fill the teeth. Devitalization of the pulp, or destroying the nerve, as it is commonly called, can be performed in different ways.

The actual cautery, or the rapid insertion of the red-hot point of an instrument, has generally been abandoned. Excision of the pulp by insinuating a delicate smooth instrument with a sharp and slightly bent point, between the pulp and the wall of the canal up to the point where the vessels enter, and then making a revolving cut, is the most speedy method. If the operation is performed dextrously, there is little or no pain given; but persons so often object to it that the methods of destroying the pulp generally adopted, are those of applying either cobalt or arsenious acid. Of these two methods the latter is most in vogue. For this purpose the arsenious acid, or white arsenic, is generally mixed into a paste with acetate of morphia and creasote The arsenious acid in its action irritates and increases the circulation of the pulp to the point of strangulation and stagnation. Its dilution and thorough effect is accomplished by means of the morphia, while both the morphia and the creasote obtund the sensibility of the nervous matter which would otherwise be greatly exalted by the pressure of the increased circulation. Quite a number of dentists oppose the use of arsenious acid on the ground of the danger of its being absorbed and destroying the investing membrane of the tooth and parts beyond, and use cobalt instead, claiming that it is not so dangerous an agent, although its efficacy depends upon the arsenic contained.

For my part, I do not admit the liability of the occurrence of such accidents where proper care is used in its introduction and in securing the paste in the cavity; although there is no doubt that such results might happen from mismanagement. Certain it is that I never have seen a case of injury to surrounding parts occurring from its use when properly applied, and many others of many years' experience testify to the same thing. The cavity should be thoroughly dry and a portion of the paste on cotton applied directly to the point, and the whole covered with some substance to preclude the possibility of its escape. Amalgam, or oxy-chloride of zinc filling, I have found the best. A filling of cotton dipped in sandarac varnish is also much used. The quantity of paste used need not be larger in size than half a mustard-seed, and it is safer to remove it in twenty-four hours, although some of the best dentists have experimented by leaving it in a cavity for weeks without any bad result. Frequently the arsenical paste can be pricked gradually into the pulp, and the contents of the canal removed without pain, while the patient remains in the dental chair.

13

Much judgment is often required in deciding as to the propriety of making such an application to the temporary teeth. As has been seen, at certain periods the roots are more or less absorbed to allow the advance of the permanent teeth. The application at these periods would be very injudicious, as the absorption of the arsenious acid through the wide ends of the canals might produce all the evil results that the worst enemies of arsenic claim. To relieve the pain of exposed pulps in temporary teeth at these times, and to avoid the evils following too early extraction, every remedy should be resorted to. Dr. Garretson gives an excellent formula, which may be copied and sent to an apothecary:

"℞   Creasotum, ...   gtt. vi.
     Tinct. Iodinii,   .   .   .   f ʒj.
     Aqua Plumbi, ...   f ʒss.
     Chloroform, ...
     Tinct. Opii, āā .   .   .   .   . f ʒ."

PULP NODULES.

FROM some derangement of the function of the dental pulp, either during the formation of the teeth, or on account of subsequent irritation, irregular, detached masses of dentine are occasionally formed and occupy various positions in the pulp chamber.

They are generally nodular, kidney shaped, or spicular. Frequently they are productive of no irritation, while at other times they give rise to the most violent kind of toothache, which is mistaken for neuralgia on account of the flitting character of the pain, and the different parts affected. It is a very hard matter to decide whether pulp nodules exist or not, the teeth being of perfectly healthy appearance as far as the influence of their presence is concerned; but it is warrantable to drill into the teeth for them, in cases of aggravated odontalgia, which the most complete investigation can not trace to any other cause. It has been said that teeth so affected have a peculiarly uneasy sensation upon scratching them with the finger nail, and give no pain upon pressure, but do upon striking them. If the nodules prevent the access of arsenical paste to the pulp, when applied in the opening made in the crown, a small hole can be drilled through the root into the pulp canal.

PERIODONTITIS.

This is inflammation of the periodonteum or the enveloping membrane of the root, and constitutes one of the most excruciating forms of toothache, as can be imagined when we consider that the inflamed membrane is confined closely between the hard tooth on one side and the unyielding alveolar process on the other. The sympathetic pain is far greater than that arising from an exposed pulp; other parts of the mouth, the face, eyes, ears, temples, etc., and even the neck and arms being sometimes affected to such an extent, that the real source of the trouble is overlooked. Constitutional disturbances, such as headache, fever's'ness, and constipation, are common. The inflammation sometimes extends to the tonsils and the muscles of the throat and neck. Lock-jaw has been known to result, and the death of considerable portions of the jaws. The disease begins by dull pain about the root of the tooth, with a desire to work it with the finger or with the opposite teeth. Afterward the pain becomes acute and pulsating; the tooth becomes elongated by the membrane becoming engorged, and pushing it partly from its socket; the striking of the tooth, or the pressure of the opposite teeth gives intense pain. The gum becomes red and more or less swollen. The most common causes of periodontitis are those which follow. Blows, etc., accumulation of tartar, irritation of badly fitted clasps or plates, loose roots, crowded and irregular teeth, inflammation of the pulp, dead and decomposing pulp, arsenic escaping from a cavity, and inflammation of neighboring parts may produce it. It may result from dental manipulations; as from too hard malleting, the pushing of filling material through the opening at the apex of the root, the breaking off of probes in the root canal, from putting so much filling in cavities that correct articulation is prevented and the tooth receives too much pressure, from hastily wedging apart the teeth preparatory to filling, and from rubber rings, used in regulating, slipping under the gum and remaining unseen.

The action of mercury taken internally, or absorbed from large amalgam fillings, may cause it.

Recession of the gums exposing the cementum, or the sharp edges of cavities of decay beneath the gum, may induce periodontitis. Unnatural antagonism of the teeth caused by the irregularity resulting from extraction, or no antagonism at all, may cause it. Dr. Watson, in his Practice of Physic, relates a case of blindness in an eye and suppuration of the parts around it, attributable to inflammation of the investing membrane of the root of a tooth.

The patient after much suffering presented himself to a surgeon for the purpose of having the eye cut out, but he quickly recovered after the extraction of a molar tooth, in one root of which a wooden tooth-pick had been broken off and extended a little distance beyond the apex of the root. I once saw a violent case of periodontitis that was caused by a portion of the septa of an apple core becoming buried in the alveolus of a molar tooth and firmly wedged between one of its roots and the alveolar process.

The methods of treatment are of course various, and mostly come in the province of the dental physician; but it will not be amiss to allude to their general character. Removing the cause, lancing the gums, and painting them with equal parts of tincture of iodine and aconite root, is generally the first treatment employed. Then counter-irritation, leeches, hot foot-baths, purgation, quiet, elevation of the head and the retention of something between the other teeth to prevent antagonism, are indicated.

Cooling mouth-washes are very beneficial. Chlorate of potash, one part to sixteen of water, is excellent for holding in the mouth, and a teaspoonful may be swallowed every hour or so. If it happens that it is impossible to allay the inflammation after a fair trial, then suppuration should be encouraged by painting the gums frequently with capsicum and chloroform, or with cantharidal collodion, or by applying a roasted fig or raisin. Poultices should never be applied to the outside of the face, for if the abscess should point and break there, a permanent and unsightly scar might result.

ALVEOLAR ABSCESS.

If the inflammation of periodontitis is not subdued by proper treatment, it passes on to the formation of pus, which lifts the membrane from the root, and thus forms the sac so often seen when teeth so affected are extracted. As the matter accumulates, the pressure produces absorption of that portion of the bone and the enveloping soft parts which offer the least resistance, until there is an opening made for the escape of the pus.

This opening, when formed in the gum, as it usually is, is called a gum-boil; but it sometimes happens that it is made at some distant point, in the nasal cavity, through the roof of the mouth, through the cheek, underneath the lower jaw, low down in the neck, or at some other point.

Openings discharging pus, occurring in such remote localities, are often very confusing and lead to great mistakes in treatment; especially as a casual examination of the mouth frequently detects nothing wrong with the teeth. But it must be remembered that dead pulps, a prominent cause of alveolar abscess, sometimes exist without any external decay or any noticeable discoloration of the teeth. In such cases, by holding a small mirror back of the tooth and reflecting light against it, an opaque appearance is observable that does not exist in a tooth with a living pulp.

A wisdom-tooth that does not erupt for want of room may be the cause. A broken piece of root left in the socket at a previous extraction, hidden by the gum and not known by the patient, may be the cause of such purulent discharge. The other causes of alveolar abscess have been sufficiently noticed in the enumeration of those which are capable of producing an attack of periodontitis. The throbbing pain that accompanies the formation of alveolar abscess, is often of the most agonizing nature until the escape of the matter, when sudden relief comes; therefore the propriety of hastening suppuration by the applications mentioned in the last chapter, as soon as ultimate abscess is found to be inevitable. After the pus has escaped, the opening generally heals in a few days, but abscess is very liable to recur at some future time, unless the tooth is properly treated and filled; and even then its prevention is not certain, although a well-performed operation is very often successful. Sometimes the abscess settles down into a chronic form, and there is a slight but continued oozing of pus, in which case longer treatment is required.

Teeth that have no antagonists are occasionally pushed from their sockets sufficiently to allow the escape of the matter around their necks. Among the worst effects of alveolar abscess may be mentioned necrosis of the teeth, and loss of several neighboring processes, or even of considerable portions of the jaw. Abscesses connected with children's temporary teeth are peculiarly dangerous in this respect. Chronic abscess, by the constant discharge of pus into the mouth, vitiates its fluids, thus injuring the teeth and deranging the general system. In the treatment of alveolar abscess the value of the affected tooth should be considered; if an old root or an isolated tooth it should be extracted. If it is desirable to save it, the pulp canal should be cleaned out, and the fistulous opening continuous with it injected with diluted creasote, iodine, phenol sodique, or some other curative agent. Cutting through the gum and alveolar process to the root, and destroying the sac, is a method often resorted to with success. In depraved conditions of the system general medical treatment is often necessary.

After the tooth is brought to a healthy condition, the root and the crown cavity should be filled as already described. As before mentioned, the abscess should never be allowed to break anywhere on the face, even if it can not be prevented except by very free lancing on the inside of the cheeks. Otherwise a permanent fistulous opening and disfigurement might result. Of course if such an accident should occur, the dental or the general surgeon would be able to restore the parts partially or entirely, but it is best to avoid the necessity of a surgical operation.

DECOMPOSITION IN THE PULP CAVITY.

OCCASIONALLY it happens that a greater or less portion of the pulp loses its vitality, the inflammation stopping short of periodontitis and alveolar abscess.

The dead portion decomposes, forming pus and mephitic gas; if these are prevented from escaping by a sound crown, a filling, impervious dentine or impacted food, they irritate the portion of living pulp at the extremity of the canal. The odontalgia arising is usually very severe and assumes a neuralgic form.

The gas arising from the putrefaction of food which becomes condensed in the first portion of the canal while there is some vitality in the other part, produces the same effect. This condition of affairs often comes about when an old filling, that has caused by its presence the destruction of a part of the pulp, drops out and the patient fails to have it renewed; also, where the frequent application of creasote for the relief of toothache has caused such partial devitalization, and the tooth has not been filled afterward.

The treatment is to clean out the pulp cavity to the point of vitality, and fill after all inflammation is subdued. When such cases are taken in time, the operation is more than ordinarily successful compared with other pulp complications, on account of the distance existing between the body of the filling and the point of sensitiveness. Sometimes the decomposed matter is absorbed into the tubules of the dentine, discoloring the tooth, and trouble is prevented for a long time.

FUNGOUS PULP, ETC.

In very large cavities of decay, involving the exposure of the pulp, it sometimes occurs that the pulp fails to take on acute inflammation, the irritation of external agents only succeeding in exciting enlargement. The fungous growth may be so large as to fill the cavity; the larger it is the less sensitiveness and the more hemorrhage upon pricking.

The smaller growths are often very sensitive. Sometimes when severely wounded by the contact of food in mastication, pain occurs of greater or less duration. The rational treatment would be to relieve sensitiveness by creasote, promote absorption by iodine, or cut out the growth and destroy the pulp in the canal, and afterward fill; but I have succeeded in effecting a cure by cutting away the tumor, stopping the bleeding in a few minutes, capping and permanently filling. At times, what appears to be a fungous pulp, will be found on close investigation to be a fungous growth of the gum, entering an opening in the neck of the tooth, the sharp edges of which cause the irritation that produces the enlargement.

The application of arsenical paste in such a case would be very injurious, so great care should be observed in ascertaining of what the growth really consists.

If the tumor proceeds from the investing membrane of the root, extraction is generally necessary.

DENTAL EXOSTOSIS.

THIS is the name given to the enlargement of the roots of the teeth, produced by the deposit of new osseous material. The extraneous substance may be deposited with some regularity about the circumference of the roots; but generally it is in the form of bulbs or protuberances of various sizes. The deposit is occasionally so abundant that the alveolar partitions are absorbed, and the roots of different teeth inseparably joined.

This abnormal growth may result from various causes which irritate the membrane sufficiently to cause it to throw out more osseous matter, or it may occur on account of some inexplicable constitutional peculiarity. The disease is not confined to any particular condition of the affected teeth, for the crowns may be perfectly sound, decayed slightly or much, or entirely gone. The irritating causes to which exostosis has generally been traced are: unnatural antagonism of the teeth; mechanical injuries from accidents; hard usage, such as cracking nuts, etc.; deposition of tartar; protruding fillings; the conduction of hot and cold impressions by fillings; fractures in attempts to extract; loose teeth; grinding of the teeth; imperfectly fitted clasps and plates; cavities encroaching on the cementum, etc.

The disease is generally very slow in its development, the pain at first being slight, or only an uncomfortable feeling about the roots being present; in the latter stages, however, the suffering is often unbearable and peculiarly aggravating on account of its neuralgic character disguising its real location.

In Harris' Dental Surgery allusion is made to the case of dental exostosis which came under the observation of the celebrated Fox. The subject, a young lady, at the time she presented herself to him, "had suffered so much and so long, that the palpebræ of one eye had been closed for near two months, and the secretion of saliva had, for some time, been so copious that it flowed from her mouth whenever opened. She had tried every remedy science and skill could suggest, without experiencing any permanent benefit, and was only relieved from her suffering by the extraction of every one of her teeth." The only remedy in the advanced stages is extraction; but there is no doubt that if the disease should be suspected in its incipient state, it could often be prevented by the treatment applicable to periodontitis. Even when extraction is decided upon, it is often a matter of great difficulty, depending upon the manner in which the osseous material has been deposited. Sometimes it is an absolute impossibility without first cutting away the alveolar process to the extremity of the root.

EXPOSED CEMENTUM.

The cementum when divested of its natural coverings, the alveolar process, and the superimposed gum, is exquisitely sensitive. There are several methods whereby this exposure may be produced: Inflammation, and subsequent recession of the gums, occasioned by vitiated fluids, or any local or constitutional cause; deposits of different kinds of tartar; loose or irregularly placed teeth, and the pressing away of the gums by artificial partial plates. When teeth have lost their antagonists, there is usually an effort of nature to remove them from their sockets, thus lifting the cementum from its protective surroundings. Where no particular cause is found to exist, many attribute the recession of the gums to premature old age exhibiting itself in this one location at least, recognizing the fact that the teeth of aged people are generally gotten rid of in this way. Such a supposition does not seem any more unreasonable than to attribute the early appearance of gray hairs to the same cause.

The success attending the treatment of exposed cementum arising from the effects of the saliva, or from constitutional causes, is not very encouraging as far as permanent relief from annoyance is concerned. Acids and alkalies are used respectively to correct alkalinity and acidity. Elongating teeth require artificial antagonists. Pressing plates should be discarded for those raised a little from the gums where they surround the teeth. Loose teeth should be supported and irregular ones regulated. Tartar should be removed and kept from again accumulating. Conjointly, various obtunding agents may be used.

DENTAL NECROSIS.

WHEN from any cause both the pulp and the peridentium of the tooth are destroyed, or in other words, when both the external and the internal sustenance are cut off, the tooth is said to be entirely dead or necrosed. Its color then changes, the discoloration varying from a yellowish hue to nearly black, depending much upon the manner of its death, the capacity of absorption of the decomposed matter by the dentinal tubes, and whether or not a cavity exists in the tooth.

A necrosed tooth is further distinguished by its being more or less elongated, and by the gums not clinging to it when it is worked back and forth by the fingers.

When any of the other osseous structures of the body are affected with necrosis, nature refuses to tolerate the dead portions, and they are thrown off, or exfoliated; but necrosed teeth are often, where the constitutional conditions are favorable, permitted to remain in position a long time. This is accounted for by the fact that the teeth are not really part and parcel of the surrounding bone, but are held somewhat separated from it by sockets so shaped as to mechanically retain the teeth in position until any inflammation arising from their presence, if not too violent, has exhausted itself.

During the activity of the causes that produce the necrosis, and during the efforts of nature to rid herself of the offending tooth, various degrees of pain are felt, from very slight to very severe. Necrosis of the teeth may be produced by anything that has elsewhere been seen to be capable of causing inflammation and death of the pulp, these extending to the peridentium; by the action of certain medicinal agents, and through lack of sufficient nutrition, as occurs sometimes in the debilitated conditions following wasting fevers, etc.

Threatened necrosis is to be combated by the same general and local treatment that has been advised for inflammation of the pulp and periodontitis. After it has occurred, the discolored teeth can often be bleached and filled, with the prospect of saving them for a considerable time.

Before leaving this subject, it may be well to bestow passing notice upon those forms of necrosis involving the alveolar processes, or more or less of the jaw bones; but the general surgeon is more frequently consulted about these cases than the dentist. The death of the periosteum, or the membrane which affords vitality to the bones, causes the death of those portions which are nourished by it. Such necrosis often happens from accidents of various kinds; from the extent of inflammation from diseased teeth; from crowded wisdom-teeth; from attacks of such diseases as small-pox, measles and scarlet-fever; from the administration of mercury and exposure to phosphorus; from scrofulous and other taints of the system. The symptoms at first are hardly distinguishable from those attending inflammation about the roots of the teeth, but as the disease manifests itself, there is no mistaking the extent, the purple, glazed appearance and pain of the swelling, the fistulous openings and the fetid discharge.

The treatment essentially consists of the removal of the dead bone, the administration of tonic medicines, and the local application of washes for stimulation and purification.

SYMPATHY—NEURALGIA.

No matter what lines of demarkation may be drawn by scientific men between ordinary, sympathetic and neuralgic pains, it is evident that these distinctions are not comprehended by the people nor generally observed by the physiologically educated. Probably the simplest definitions that can be given are the following. Ordinary pain proceeds from local irritation, being readily traced to its seat and causing disagreeable sensations nowhere else. The term sympathetic pain should probably be confined to that which experience teaches, exists in certain parts while other parts are the ones really irritated, so frequently as to be regarded a symptom of the distant irritation; thus pain in the shoulder generally accompanies irritation of the liver; pain in the left arm is associated with certain diseases of the heart; and pain in sound teeth may occur from pregnancy, rheumatism, gout, or from other teeth that are diseased.

Neuralgia, properly speaking, means an affection of the trunk of a nerve, the pain appearing to proceed along its course and into its branches of termination.

Even the names themselves are very unsatisfactory, for neuralgia is derived from Greek words meaning nerve-pain; therefore any pain might be called neuralgia, as it is irritation of the nerves that produces the sensation. Then it is not very comforting to the patient who has been suffering the raging pain of toothache, rendered somewhat more bearable by the *sympathy* of kind friends at home, to go to the *sympathetic* dentist and there be informed that *sympathy* is the cause of all his troubles. He might naturally conclude that he had received enough of it, and be excused for becoming irritable at any further *sympathy* being evinced by commiserating friends.

The phenomena connected with the nervous system are more wonderful and incomprehensible than any others observed in the animal organism, and but few of them are fully explained by the various theories concerning the nature of nervous substance and the manner of the transmission of nervous impressions. It will be most suitable for our purpose to consider the brain and the spinal marrow as batteries generating animal electricity; then to regard the twelve cranial and the thirty-one spinal nerves as conducting wires by which motion and sensation are respectively conveyed to and from every part of the body; and lastly to consider the great sympathetic nerve, with its independent generating ganglia and various cords, as the means of establishing nervous communication between all of the different portions of the body.

By this theory the *possibility* of the conveyance of sympathetic and neuralgic painful impressions is made manifest; but *why* the impressions should be so conveyed to the various parts of this intricately woven web of nervous tissue, interfering with their harmonious action, is a mystery never to be explained.

> "Like warp and woof, * * * *
> Are woven fast,
> Linked in sympathy like the keys
> Of an organ vast;
> Pluck one thread and the web ye mar,
> Break but one
> Of a thousand keys, and the paining jar
> Through all will run."

Only those that have tried know the difficulty that the dentist often has in persuading people that are not aware of the peculiarities of the nervous system, that certain teeth are the cause of violent pains that they locate elsewhere. Many persons have had tooth after tooth extracted that could have been saved, without experiencing any relief until finally the right one has been reached, possibly on the other side of the same jaw, or even in the opposite jaw.

Let us look at the few of the many recorded instances of sympathetic affections connected with diseased conditions of the teeth.

Dr. Watson, in his Practice of Physic, quotes a case of severe tic douloureux of ten years' standing, which was at last completely cured by the extraction of a decayed tooth.

Dr. Harris gives a case of a gentleman afflicted with the gout for many years, and who was forewarned of the approach of the attacks by the occurrence of toothache which came on regularly ten or twelve days before, and which ceased as the gout symptoms came on, but returned and continued for two weeks, when these subsided. From Dr. Garretson's work, I take the following cases:

A young lady had suffered for some time with neuralgia of the face, ear and scalp; her agony was sometimes so great that she had to resort for temporary relief to the inhalation of chloroform; she had experienced no pain in any of her teeth, but all of her pain instantly disappeared upon the extraction of a carious bicuspid with an exposed pulp.

A lady aged thirty had suffered for ten years from severe neuralgia, affecting the left eyeball and left side of the head and face, the iris of the affected eye having changed from a deep and bright hazel to a dull gray. Upon the extraction of an exostosed tooth the pain left.

A woman affected with facial neuralgia was cured by the extraction of a central incisor that was sound, but somewhat elongated and slightly loose. Upon opening the tooth, an excrescence of dentine was found encroaching on the pulp.

A lady was afflicted with neuralgia of the left fore-arm from the pressure of a badly fitted lower set of artificial teeth.

A young woman suffering with wry-neck for more than six months, and whose head was drawn down nearly to the shoulder, was cured by the removal of some teeth.

A young lady suffered with neuralgic pains, first of the face and afterward of the arms, legs and nearly the whole body. Exostosed teeth were the cause; the crowns were entirely sound.

Dr. Hyde Salter was afflicted with neuralgia of the neck and arm, from a carious molar. There was no actual pain in the tooth itself, nor any tenderness in it or the adjacent gum, nor any appearance of inflammation. He was cured by the extraction of this tooth.

A lady of rank and a nun are mentioned as being attacked by facial neuralgia and toothache, owing to menstrual irregularities.

Epilepsy, catalepsy, blindness, deafness, lock-jaw, convulsions, St. Vitus' dance, etc., have been caused by diseased and crowded teeth.

It is useless to make further mention of particular cases; from those quoted it is obvious that it is not improbable that serious disturbances in almost any part of the body may arise from tooth irritation as a primary cause, and yet the teeth not be suspected; and on the other hand, that the teeth may suffer from disturbances in other parts of the system.

It will be superfluous to make any remarks concerning the treatment of such sympathetic and neuralgic pains, as that applicable to the diseases of the teeth causing such disturbances, is mentioned under the proper headings; while the treatment of the systemic conditions lies within the province of the general physician.

Such attacks are often invited by anything which debilitates the vital powers, as disease, debauchery, etc.; by anything which causes the accumulation of impurities in the blood, as bad atmosphere, miasmatic influences, etc.; and by exhausting emotions and passions.

S. D. Gross, M. D., Professor of Surgery in the Jefferson Medical College of Philadelphia, mentions a form of neuralgia of the jaw-bones which has not been described by others. The pain is located in the alveolar processes and overlying gum of jaws from which the teeth have been for some time extracted; and it is described as being very severe, coming on in paroxysms often from slight causes, such as talking, masticating, the contact of hot and cold food, mental excitement, etc. The disease appears to arise from the compression of the minute nerves distributed through the wasted alveolar process, dependent upon the encroachment of osseous matter upon the walls of the canals in which they are naturally inclosed.

He considers that the only effectual remedy is to cut out the affected alveolar process.

MISCELLANEOUS DISEASES.

ATROPHY.

THIS word, meaning defective nourishment, although not strictly appropriate as applied to the disease we are about to consider, is probably more nearly correct than any technical name we have; but the plain English, *tooth-marks*, conveys the meaning in a plainer manner. Atrophy is generally applied to a wasting away of any portion of the body, after being fully formed, on account of deficient nutrition; thus we say, "atrophy of the heart," or "atrophy of a limb," when these become dwindled in size, which is certainly not the idea to be conveyed concerning the teeth. We have seen, in a previous place, that the teeth, in reference to their formation and growth, are classed with such productions as nails. This similarity is nowhere more evident than in the present disease. The term atrophy, in dentistry, is used to denote certain marks which form abrupt contrast with the general color of the tooth, or which destroy the general evenness of the enamel by the formation of little pits, indentations, or grooves on its surface.

White, yellow, or brown spots of various sizes and irregular shapes may exist on the outer surfaces of the teeth; these do not interfere with the smoothness of the enamel, and although the teeth at these points are of soft structure and easily cut away, yet the places rarely decay if unmolested, on account of the lips keeping them constantly clean.

The little pits or depressions may be scattered here and there over the surface, or they may run together so as to form grooves. They may be shallow, affecting only the enamel, or deep, going through to the dentine. The incisors are the only teeth attacked in the great majority of cases, but occasionally others are also. Sometimes several of the teeth in one or both jaws may be so affected as to scarcely look like teeth, appearing as if they had been badly eaten and discolored by some corrosive agent.

Dental atrophy is doubtless produced by causes that interfere with the nutrition of the teeth during their formation; thus it frequently results from attacks of scarlet-fever, measles, small-pox, etc., just as the nails exhibit grooves of imperfect development from the same causes. The white and brown spots may result from slighter disturbances, as the irregular white spots in the nails do. External violence may sometimes cause them before the teeth are erupted, just as a blow over the root of the nail below the scarf-skin shows its effect afterward when the injured part, as a purple spot, is pushed forward by the growing nail.

Concerning the treatment, little need be said. If the pits are shallow and easily kept clean, no harm will arise. If they are deep, they ought to be filled as cavities of decay; if near the cutting edge of the tooth, they can often be removed by the file. In the worst cases, where filling would be impossible, and the disfigurement of the personal appearance is so great as to be a source of mortification, it is certainly justifiable to advise extraction and the insertion of artificial teeth.

ABRASION OF THE TEETH.

By this term is meant the wearing away of the cutting and grinding surfaces of the teeth. The front teeth are much more affected than the back ones, the former being sometimes worn away, even to the gums. The pulps of the teeth would, of course, be exposed in the early stages of the disease, were it not for a wonderful provision of nature by which they are stimulated to throw out new dentinal substance for their protection, while they gradually retire before the advance of the enemy. But there is a limit to this self-protection, and the pulps are generally so nearly uncovered at some period in the progress of the abrasion, that they become much irritated from mastication, hot and cold food, acids, etc. Several causes have been assigned for this wasting of the substance of the teeth; the manner of their shutting together; very hard food; acidity of some of the secretions; imperfect texture of the teeth, and excessive power of the masticatory muscles.

But I can not see that either of these is always sufficient. It is true that in the majority of cases of abrasion, the upper front teeth shut squarely upon the lower ones instead of over them; but this ought to cause the wearing away of the front teeth only until the back teeth receive all of the strain upon themselves. Although old sailors who have used hard biscuits for a great many years, usually have the crowns of their teeth much worn down, yet many persons who live on land and eat easily masticated food, have their teeth affected in the same way. If it depends upon the fluids of the mouth exerting a corrosive influence, all of the teeth ought to be affected similarly, and all parts of the teeth should be more or less acted upon.

Abraded teeth generally have the external evidences of being solidly constructed, and are comparatively free from decay. Excessive muscular power appears to be a very common feature, but many individuals who have just as much, and whose teeth shut properly, have no abrasion.

The treatment depends upon the existing circumstances. If several teeth have been lost and undue force is exerted upon the others, artificial teeth can be inserted so as to sustain the greater portion of the pressure. Sensitive dentine may receive the treatment that has been advised in another part of this work. Exposed, or nearly exposed pulps, may be devitalized and the root canals filled. Where the abraded front teeth have to be extracted, the insertion of artificial teeth is often a matter of peculiar difficulty if the other teeth are left in; for the plate and teeth require frequently so much space that the jaws are opened somewhat, which prevents the back teeth of one jaw from touching those of the opposite. Rubber plates will hardly ever do; gold or silver ones often answer well, if the teeth can be set without disfigurement so as to allow the opposite natural teeth to strike the plate only. If filing the natural teeth does not give sufficient room, it is often necessary to extract the balance of the teeth on the same jaw with the abraded ones, and insert an entire half set which can be arranged to suit any irregularities.

There is another wasting of the points of the front teeth, which leaves a space between them and the teeth of the opposite jaw, instead of being followed up and worn still further by them. Writers have incorrectly termed this "spontaneous abrasion." Abrasion means wearing away by rubbing with a sufficiently hard substance, and there is certainly no such mechanical action here. The disease doubtless arises from defective tooth material and acid fluids.

DENUDATION OF THE TEETH.

This is the name given to a slow corrosion of the enamel, and ultimately of the dentine, on the anterior faces of the teeth. It differs from pitted atrophy in that it occurs long after the eruption of the teeth, and instead of being rough in appearance, is perfectly smooth and highly polished. It sometimes forms a continuous groove across several of the teeth near the gum, just as if made by a half round file and then polished. As has been seen in the chapter on Sensitive Dentine, pain may arise after the enamel has been removed. It is probably the same thing as "spontaneous abrasion," only in a different locality. The avoidance of brushes with stiff bristles, and the use of antacid washes, are the best means to delay its progress, with the exception of filling. The latter is generally objected to on account of the number and conspicuousness of the fillings, but the good dental operator might not object to thus posting up a modest advertisement.

DISEASES OF THE ANTRUM, OR MAXILLARY SINUS.

When we consider the fact that those best acquainted with the anatomy of the human body, were, three hundred years ago, ignorant of the existence of the maxillary sinus, and that its uses have never yet been discovered, it is not so surprising that the majority of the people do not know that there is a large cavity of that name in each side of the upper jaw.

It is situated above the back teeth, the roots of the bicuspids and molars either entering it or being only slightly separated by a thin layer of bone. The floor of the orbit forms its roof, and all of its walls are quite thin. It communicates with the cavity of the nose by a small opening, and is everywhere lined by a continuation of its mucous membrane, which has its proper secretion. It is liable to the same diseases, that mucous membranes are generally, and to some others depending upon its peculiar situation. Its diseases range from those of the simplest nature that readily submit to treatment, to those of such a complicated and violent character that death alone stops their ravages.

Some simple diseases that could readily be cured by the proper early attention, may be neglected or mistreated until they baffle the skill of the dentist and physician.

Debilitated and depraved conditions of the system resulting from exhausting diseases, vicious habits, scrofulous and other taints, etc., have much to do with the character and violence of the diseases of the antrum. The presence of diseased teeth is a more common cause of trouble than all other causes combined. Inflammation often extends from diseased roots to the mucous membrane of this cavity; the character of its secretion is changed, it becomes irritating and emits an exceedingly disagreeable odor. Occasionally the passage into the nose becomes closed and the accumulated secretion distends the cavity, breaks down the weakest wall, pushing out the eye, turning aside the nose, depressing the palate, elevating the cheek, or closing the nostril. Abscesses may be formed with fistulous openings through the cheek, into the orbit, nose, etc. Ulcerations, innocent or dangerous, may occur. Tumors, from the simple and curable kind to the malignant and incurable, may grow to various sizes. Cases are recorded where they have produced death by pressing upon the brain, crowding into the throat, or by exhausting the system. Caries and necrosis may attack the walls of the cavity and associated parts, causing exfoliation of the dead portions and great disfigurement of the soft parts.

Most of the diseases of the antrum have a similar general character, such as deep-seated pain in the upper jaw, flushed cheek, offensive discharge from the nostril when the position of the head favors its gravitation into the nose, and sympathetic pain in other parts of the head. Nearly every disease has some symptom different from the rest, by which the experienced observer may distinguish it to a certainty. When some other cause is not known, the teeth ought to be carefully examined. Old roots may remain, unknown to the patient, the gums being closed over them. Teeth may have dead and putrescent pulps, and the external appearance of the tooth not be affected. But the hidden causes of the diseases of the teeth, and the methods of their detection, have been considered in another place. Diseases of the antrum occasionally are caused otherwise than by bad teeth; thus affections of the nasal passages may close the opening, and foreign substances may find entrance into the cavity. The treatment of its diseases is the same that is applicable to conditions of a similar nature occurring in other parts. Tumors must be cut out and dead bone removed. An opening for the escape of accumulated secretion and for the purpose of injection, is generally made by the extraction of one or more teeth and enlarging the alveoli. Of the many cases that have been placed on record, in which obscure troubles have been traced to diseased teeth as their origin, I select the following:

Harris gives an account of a young lady from the West Indies who was afflicted for many months with a fistulous opening under the right eye. Medical treatment availed nothing, and finally a carious molar was extracted. The operation was followed by the immediate discharge of a large quantity of thick, muddy and greenish matter, and a cure was accomplished without further treatment.

In a case reported for the Dental Cosmos by Horace Meredith White, M. D., the patient was troubled for some time by a fetid discharge from the right nostril, and heat and sense of tension in the same side of the jaw. After the extraction of a decayed molar and the escape of pus, the disease was cured.

Garretson quotes a case from Baron Haller in which a large tumor of the cheek existed. The external wall was much distended and softened, and yielded to pressure, upon the removal of which it gave a sound resembling the crushing of an egg-shell. The nose was turned to one side and the nostril was obstructed, yet the patient suffered no pain. The case was cured by the extraction of some bicuspid and molar roots and some after treatment.

In another case, a young woman had complained of a dull aching pain under the orbit for three or four months; this was attended by a gradual elevation of the plate of bone between the antrum and the eye. Blindness and a discharge from the nostril followed. Recovery took place after the removal of three roots affected with periodontitis.

RANULA.

The ducts of the submaxillary and sublingual salivary glands enter the floor of the mouth beneath the anterior portion of the tongue. Occasionally one of these becomes closed and the secretion accumulates, distending the duct and forming a tumor of a smaller or larger size. The contents may be either fluid in the early stages, or solid at a later period from the absorption of the watery portions, the mineral matter being left and forming a mass similar in consistency to the salivary calculus found on the teeth. Such swellings are sometimes so large as to push the tongue back into the throat, interfering with mastication, swallowing and enunciation.

They are at times very rapid in growth, as shown by the following case:

The patient "stated that the enlargement occurred while eating his breakfast, and that in five minutes it attained the size of 'a walnut with its bark on,' and that it prevented his opening his mouth freely. After leaving the table he rubbed it for some time, and in half an hour it was reduced to its present size. From that time the same enlargement occurred every time he ate, and without reference to what he ate. It enlarged most, however, while eating his first meal in the morning. By rubbing alone could it be reduced. Chewing tobacco seemed rather to diminish than to increase its size. It was not tender nor red, but when enlarged to its utmost, it caused a severe pain, which extended to his ear." The treatment generally adopted is to puncture the sac, let out the contents and insert into the opening a short tube with expanded ends, so as to hold it in position; or else to cut out with the scissors a portion of the sac, and follow with astringent lotions. The term ranula is not usually applied to an enlargement resulting from the closure of the duct of the parotid gland, which opens opposite the second molar tooth of the upper jaw; but I will mention that condition here, although its occurrence is rare. In the British Journal of Dental Science a case is reported of closure of the parotid duct and swelling of the cheek, caused by inflammation resulting from the ragged edge of the second molar.

INFLAMMATION OF THE GUMS.

The gums, in a healthy condition of the mouth and the general system, present a pale pink appearance; their margins taper down to thin edges, forming regular festoons around the necks of the teeth, which they embrace so closely as to aid materially in retaining them in position; their texture is quite tough, enabling them to withstand the pressure and friction of mastication, and vigorous rubbing with the brush without any pain, bleeding or injury. But from various local and constitutional causes their normal characteristics are so changed, that in fact it is quite rare to see a person possessing perfectly healthy gums.

All grades of inflammation may occur, from a slight swelling around one tooth to a tumefaction so great as to nearly cover all of them. With the different degrees, may be associated suppuration, sensitiveness so great as to prevent the mastication of anything but soft food, and hemorrhage upon the slightest touch of a tooth-pick or tooth-brush. The usual local causes of inflammation are: the use of irritating brushes, picks and powders; poorly fitting plates and clasps; the accumulation of decomposing food under unremoved artificial plates and between the natural teeth; collections of tartar or salivary calculus; irregularly placed, loose and dead teeth; irritating edges of roots and cavities of decay; ligatures and rings around the teeth for regulating, etc.; wedges placed between the teeth for separating; substances crowded underneath the gums, such as portions of metal fillings and the septa of the cores of fruit; the unskillful use of creasote, chloride of zinc, and other powerful medicines; periodontitis and several diseases of the teeth and jaws; teeth without antagonists; erupting teeth; irritating substances that sometimes exist in tobacco and in various articles of food. The most of these combine to form one great cause, which does the mischief in nineteen cases out of twenty, and that is,—lack of cleanliness and care about the mouth.

The main treatment is to remove and keep away the cause, which alone will generally effect a cure; but various healing washes may be used also.

Phenol sodique, two teaspoonsful or more to a glass of water; two drachms each of chlorate of potash and borax to four ounces of water; two teaspoonsful of chlorinated soda to a glass of water; white oak bark and water boiled together; are a few of the many washes employed for ordinary inflammation of the gums.

Dr. Harris gives two good prescriptions for "inflamed, spongy and ulcerated gums:

"℞. Powdered nutgalls, ... 2 drachms.
       Powdered Peruvian bark, . . 2 drachms.
       Powdered orris root, ... 1 drachm.
       Infusion of roses, ... 4 fluid ounces.

"The infusion to stand for a day or so upon the powders, with frequent stirring, then decant and filter.

"℞. Borax, ... 2 scruples.
       Honey, ... 1 fluid ounce.
       Sage tea, ... 4 fluid ounces.

"This is a favorite and very general domestic remedy, and will be found very soothing and healing." A solution of nitrate of silver, to be applied by the dentist to the margins of the gums, is certain and rapid in its effect.

For the inflamed gums attending periodontitis, one of the best washes is:

R. Chlorate of potash, ... 4 drachms.
    Water, ... 8 fluid ounces.
    Laudanum, ... 2 fluid drachms.

A teaspoonful of this should be taken into the mouth every half hour and held for some minutes so as to submerge the inflamed gum, and then spit out. Certain morbid growths of the gums should be removed by the knife.

Different diseases, affecting the system generally, but having an especial local manifestation in the gums, should receive general medical treatment; among these may be mentioned scurvy and the mercurial disease. Local treatment in conjunction should not be omitted, however.

More might be said concerning the different affections of the gums, but they are mentioned incidentally in other places in this volume.

TUMORS.

The maxillary bones and the parts in immediate connection with them, are peculiarly liable to these morbid enlargements. They may be like bone, flesh or cartilage in consistence; of small or immense proportions; of slow or rapid growth; painless or excessively painful; of various shades of color, from pale to purple. They may be smooth and of symmetrical proportions, or they may be rough and of very irregular form; attached by either a broad or a stem-like base. Some occur only at certain periods of life, others at any time. The state of the patient's health may be not at all affected for years, or it may be disturbed at the earliest periods. Some are readily cured by removal and treatment, while others persistently return and ultimately carry the sufferer to the grave. To give a description of the various kinds of tumors and their symptoms would be a task too tedious. Some are so complicated that the most experienced doctors find themselves bewildered. This advice is always good, however: the patient should never permit a tumor to exist without presenting himself to a physician, dentist or surgeon, not being indifferent on account of its slow progress and mild appearance; on the other hand he should not be greatly frightened at more alarming symptoms.

Frequently it happens that small tumors, which at first could be readily removed by a simple operation, are neglected until a considerable portion of the jaw has to be lost. Tumors of the jaws and gums are more frequently traced to diseased teeth than any other cause, their magnitude and character depending much of course upon constitutional peculiarities.

The sharp edges of a decayed place, or of a root, may irritate the gums or the membrane covering the root or the alveolar process to an increased action, that results in a morbid growth.

Crowded teeth and salivary calculus may exert the same influence. Unerupted teeth may remain for some time incased somewhere in the bony structure of the jaws without producing trouble, and then become the cause of a tumor. The simple extraction of a tooth will sometimes result in a cure; at others, more or less of the jaw has to be removed. Many simple tumors of the gums can be removed by a simple cut of the knife, or by the gradual contraction of ligatures; the latter method is preferable, when they can be made to operate sufficiently low, on account of the lessened hemorrhage.

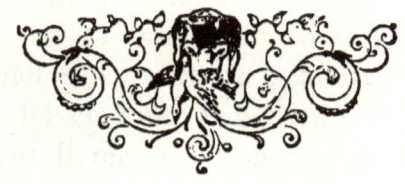

THIRD DENTITION.

MORE for the sake of gratifying the curiosity of those who may take an interest in anomalies than for any practical good, I will mention the fact that nature does occasionally, late in life, supply the toothless mouth with a new set of teeth. Many writers, who had not themselves seen such cases, have refused to believe them possible, but evidence from different sources has accumulated to such an extent, that there can no longer be any doubt. Not stopping to refer to the reported cases of remote times, which we might justly hesitate to believe, we will confine ourselves to the consideration of a few of the well-authenticated modern instances. Sinclair says: "I once saw an old man, named James Donald, who had got new teeth, which I had an opportunity personally of examining. They appeared to be much softer than teeth usually are and not fit to do the same service; and, on the whole, I was disposed to consider them as an imperfect substitute."

In Harris' Dental Surgery is an extract of a letter from a professional friend, Dr. J. D. McCabe:

"I have just seen a case of third dentition. The subject of this 'playful freak of nature,' as Dr. Good styles it, is now in his seventy-eighth year, and, as he playfully remarked, 'is just cutting his teeth.' There are eleven cut, five in the upper, and six in the lower jaw. Their appearance is that of bone, extremely rough, without any coating or enamel, and of a dingy brown color."

"Sometimes these teeth are produced with wonderful rapidity; but in such cases, with very great pain, from the callosity of the gums, through which they have to force themselves. The Edinburgh Medical Commentaries supply us with an instance of this kind. The individual was in his sixty-first year and altogether toothless. At this time his gums and jaw-bones became painful, and the pain was at length excruciating. But, within the space of twenty-one days from its commencement, both jaws were furnished with a new set of teeth, complete in number."

Such teeth are generally of poor quality, and often without well-formed roots and without sockets to retain them. In Harris' work, I find the following passage: "It is said that the efforts made by nature, for the production of a third complete set of teeth, are so great that they exhaust the remaining energies of the system; and, as a consequence, that occurrences of this kind are generally soon followed by death." But the third dentition of the grandfather of Dr. Slare (mentioned elsewhere), appears to present quite an exception to this rule of failing energy; he got his third set at eighty-five years of age and "remained in good health and strength to the one hundreth year of his age, and even then died in consequence of fullness of blood."

The teeth must have been of fair quality, also, to have lasted him fifteen years. Numerous instances have occurred in which one or two particular teeth of the second set have been replaced with new ones, and Harris even gives a case in which there were four eruptions of a certain central incisor.

SUPERNUMERARY TEETH.

IT is not very uncommon to see in the mouth a certain little tooth of stunted growth, over and above the number usually found in the jaws. Most frequently such teeth are in the front part of the upper jaw, between and rather back of the central incisors, and have cone shaped crowns. When they are found back in the jaw, they generally appear like dwarf bicuspids or stunted wisdom teeth. Dr. Harris says, however, that he has seen cases, in both jaws, in which there were too many incisors, and yet the supernumerary ones could not be distinguished, so close was their similarity to the others. Supernumerary teeth should always be extracted, when they occasion any disfigurement or irregularity. The following is a case of my own: A lad aged seventeen presented himself with five teeth in the space between the two eye-teeth. Four of these were the proper central and lateral incisors, and the other was a conical supernumerary. He informed me that a short time before he had a similar conical tooth extracted from the same space.

His incisors being decayed nearly away, they were extracted for the purpose of inserting artificial teeth. Soon after this, a peculiarly dwarfed and twisted tooth erupted and was extracted. On its root was a notch where the root of the lateral incisor had caught it, keeping it from erupting sooner. Thus it is seen that there were seven teeth in the space intended for four.

UNITED TEETH.

FAR back in history we have accounts of the occasional union of the teeth. Herodotus says that there was found on the field of the battle of Platæa "a skull without any seam, made entirely of a single bone; likewise a jaw, both the upper bone and the under, wherein all the teeth front and back, were joined together and made of one bone." Pyrrhus, king of Epirus, and a son of Prusias, king of Bithynia, are said to have had teeth of the same description.

When we consider that no such case of general union of the teeth has been found in modern times, we can be excused for incredulity concerning the statements; but the union of two of the teeth has been seen so frequently as to almost take away the novelty. Within the last month, I saw a case of the osseous union of the crowns of the lower right lateral and cuspid. Anteriorly there was presented a broad surface without division; while posteriorly there was the mark of separation. Cases have occurred in extracting teeth, in which adjoining teeth have been unintentionally removed, the roots being united while the crowns were separated.

EXTRACTING.

So many allusions have been made incidentally to the circumstances which render the extraction of teeth advisable or necessary, that it will be useless to particularize here.

With the exception of temporary teeth that require removal, irregular teeth, supernumerary teeth, and crowded wisdom-teeth, cases calling for extraction, would be very rare indeed, if people would learn to take care of their mouths and have the proper preservative dental operations performed. But as people will neglect their teeth until they have become affected with incurable diseases,—or if curable, they are not able or not willing to have them treated and filled,—extraction is such a commonly performed operation, that it will be well to speak of it further.

It is an operation that is almost universally dreaded, and many will suffer weeks of pain, lose night after night of sleep and hour after hour from business, rather than submit to it. I have seen the scarred hero of many battles cry like a child when called upon to have a tooth extracted.

Considering the prevailing aversion to the operation and the many accidents that happen when it is intrusted to rough and inexperienced hands, it is truly surprising to see the class of operators frequently allowed to perform it. The extraction of a tooth is often so simple an operation, it is true, that one that has never had a forceps in his hand before, can accomplish it; but cases are constantly presenting themselves that require intelligent employment of properly shaped instruments, the application of the necessary power in the right direction, an intimate knowledge of the anatomy of the parts and the anomalous shapes frequently occurring in the teeth. Strength is not the only thing necessary. A large, muscular man may seize a forceps in both hands, shut his eyes, and snap off the crown of a firmly set molar at a single jerk; whereas a man of much less brute strength, might with one hand, open eyes, careful motions and skillful management, bring the entire tooth safely away.

In Harris' Dental Surgery are quoted two cases to show how serious a thing the extraction of a tooth may turn out to be. They are so similar that it will be sufficient to mention one of them. The roots of the tooth (a molar) " were greatly bifurcated and dove-tailed into the jaw, and would not pass perpendicularly out, though a slight lateral motion would have moved them instantly. The jaw proved too weak to support the monstrous pull upon it, and gave way between the second and first molars, and with it came both the anterior and posterior plates of the antrum. The broken portion extended to the spongy bones of the nose, and terminated at the lower edge of the socket of the left front incisor, containing six sound teeth. The soft parts were cut away with a knife. A severe hemorrhage ensued, but the patient soon recovered, though with excessive deformity of his face and mouth."

Few people of our times consider how thankful they ought to be for the many improvements in instruments and the skill in their management, that have taken place. Ambrose Paré, "the father of French surgery," was so much afraid of accidents in extracting, that he always separated the tooth to be operated upon from the rest with a file. And in enjoining care in the use of the "tooth-mullets," or pincers, of the period, he said: "Unless the person knows readily and cunningly how to use them, he can scarcely so carry himself but that he will force out three teeth at once." The most of the serious accidents in extracting that have occurred in recent times, have been from the use of the "tooth-key," which may be described as an instrument capable of exerting power enough to tear out the side of a house, but which is often applied to the extraction of a tooth, which it is fully competent to remove together with any neighboring teeth, or large portions of jaw that may stand in the way. The tooth-key was used almost exclusively for about fifty years, but has fortunately been entirely abandoned, except by a few old fogy operators that still cling to the friend of their youth. In its place we have forceps of various shapes, and screws and elevators for roots; but accidents still occur frequently enough to make it advisable to intrust the extraction of teeth only to competent hands. A glance at the chapter describing the permanent teeth will show the comparative ease and difficulty attending the extraction of each. Generally, the wisdom-teeth, or third molars, are the easiest pulled; next, the incisors above and below; then, the bicuspids above and the cuspids and bicuspids below; next, the cuspids, or eye-teeth, above; then, the first and second molars below; and lastly, the first and second molars above. But there are many exceptions; the roots of any of the teeth may be curved or exostosed; the roots of the molars may approach one another so as to grasp a portion of the bony process, or diverge to such an extent as to not admit of passage between the adjoining teeth.

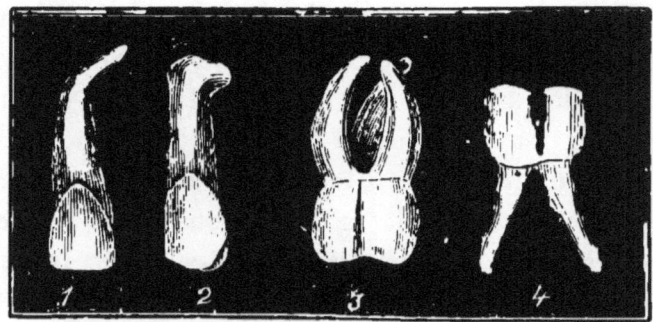

In such cases it is sometimes impossible to extract them without breaking, and the dentist is accused unjustly of awkwardness. There are several erroneous ideas engrafted in the minds of many people, that never can be eradicated until they are better educated. Some hold on tenaciously to old "eye-teeth," although they may disfigure them, or render the nice adjustment of artificial teeth impossible, because they think that to remove them will injure the eyes. I would inform those having such crotchets that these teeth are so named because the roots are long and point toward the eye, and not because there is any connection; it would be just as sensible to object to having "wisdom-teeth" extracted through fear of losing wisdom, or the "stomach-teeth" on account of injuring the stomach. Many think that the extraction of old roots is far more painful than any others, and suffer their mouths to remain in a disgusting condition for years, rather than have them removed. They are generally very easy to extract when they emerge from the gums enough to allow taking hold of them, and often are not difficult, when entirely covered by the gums. There is always an effort of nature to get rid of such old roots, and generally the process of absorption has progressed so far, that the dentist is met more than half way. Many patients, ignorant of the anatomy of the mouth, make unpleasant scenes in a dental office by declaring that roots have been left in, when the dentist knows he has removed them.

The mistake arises from feeling the bony sockets and the septa between them. The dentist ought to know, because he is aware when he has extracted the proper number of roots, and knows by the appearance of each root whether it is entire or not; but occasionally no argument will succeed in convincing the patient, and he goes to some less honorable dentist, who humors his notion for the sake of a fee or to gain his influence, and takes out a piece of the process and calls it a root.

The patient should be properly educated concerning the anatomy of the teeth, and in case of doubt should see the extracted teeth himself; thus all trouble would be avoided.

Lancing the gums is an operation that should always precede that of extracting the teeth. A great many individuals refuse to have it done, believing it to be more painful than pulling.

If the lance is sharp, it generally does not hurt at all. It facilitates the labor of extraction by severing the attachment to the gums, and to the reflected fibrous portion of the membrane of the root that embraces the neck of the tooth. Sometimes severe laceration of the gums occurs from neglect to lance.

Frequently patients circulate a report that a certain dentist has broken the jaw, when in fact there has only been a portion of the alveolar process that has given away. It is sometimes unavoidable, and generally results in no harm, only anticipating, in reality, the operation of nature in removing the processes by absorption. It is this absorption of the processes that causes the falling away of the gums after extraction. The question is often asked as to the advisability of extracting teeth during the latter months of pregnancy. It is certainly not good practice, and every means should be tried to allay pain without resorting to it. The system at such times is peculiarly susceptible to the influence of shocks of various kinds; besides miscarriage, etc., are liable enough to happen at any time, and although the extraction of a tooth might not really be the cause of the trouble, yet there would be a distressing uncertainty. Where the agony of toothache is long continued and unendurable, refusing to submit to treatment, there is no doubt that the fear of the prostrated condition of the body for the final trial, is a sufficient reason for running the risk of having teeth extracted.

In cases of violent inflammation about the teeth, abscess threatened or forming, it is often advisable to reduce the inflammation before extracting, on account of the danger of hemorrhage, or of taking cold. In greatly debilitated states of the system, or in states of violent excitement, extraction of teeth is not to be recommended.

HEMORRHAGE.

BLEEDING inside of the mouth ordinarily arises from only four causes: from brushing and picking the teeth, or spontaneously, when the gums are inflamed, and following the operations of removing tartar, lancing the gums, and extraction. The first two of these have been sufficiently noticed under "Inflammation of the Gums," and "Salivary Calculus, or Tartar." As we have seen, excessive bleeding may sometimes happen after cutting children's gums during first dentition.

In such cases, a piece of muslin, half an inch square or less, may be moistened and dipped into pulverized alum or tannin, and then held for some time against the incision by the finger of the parent; or a little clean cobweb may be retained in position by pressure.

If such simple means do not succeed, either from the unmanageability of the child, or the failure of the application, a dentist should be consulted. Sometimes a bandage has to be applied, which requires considerable skill in its adjustment. If the case is at all obstinate, internal treatment should be resorted to. In the great majority of cases there is but little hemorrhage after extraction; in fact, it is generally preferable to encourage bleeding by using warm water in the mouth, rather than to arrest it.

But occasionally it happens that the hemorrhage is alarming, and demands energetic treatment to control it, and in a few instances persons have bled to death. The object is to form a firm clot in the torn extremities of the bleeding vessels.

This can nearly always be accomplished by an observance of the following directions. Several small pledgets of cotton should be saturated with solution of persulphate of iron or tincture of nut-galls, or moistened and dipped into powdered alum or tannin, and then pressed tightly into the socket of the extracted tooth, so as to fill it up to the margin of the gum. Over this quite a large piece of cotton should be placed, so that the jaws will press tightly upon it when approximated, and yet remain separated enough to allow the saliva to run out. It should then be held in this position for an hour or more. No muscular effort should be made to spit, but the saliva should be allowed to escape by simply holding the mouth over the spittoon. When the bleeding has been stopped for some time the large piece of cotton should be removed, but that in the alveolus should not be disturbed for a day or more.

Active exercise should be avoided, and the head kept elevated. A warm foot-bath is valuable in conjunction, as it invites blood to the lower extremities. Compression is the main thing, and will often stop hemorrhage without the use of astringents, but it makes it more certain to add them. Various other applications are in the hands of the dentist, but the above mentioned are about the most available for the patient to use himself. Pledgets of cobweb applied in the manner described for the cotton pledgets, I have never known to fail.

If a tendency to hemorrhage is known to exist by previous experience, or suspected from its occurrence in other members of the same family, constitutional treatment should be employed for some days previous to the operation of extracting.

DISLOCATION OF THE LOWER JAW.

THIS is an accident that occurs occasionally from opening the mouth too wide in gaping, during the extraction of teeth, from forcing large bodies into the mouth, and from blows received when the mouth is open, etc.

A glance at any book of anatomy, showing the articulation of the jaws, will explain how the accident may occur by the condyles slipping out of the depression in which they play. The dislocation is readily recognized by the protrusion of the jaw either directly forward or partially to one side, according to whether one or both condyles have slipped out; the mouth furthermore remains wide open, and there is much pain.

As the accident might happen at a time when professional help could not be readily obtained, I will mention the manner in which the jaw is generally easily returned to its place. The patient should take both hands, and placing the fingers upon the back teeth of each side, pull with force the jaw downward and backward, while an assistant should push the chin upward, and at the same time hold a block, or the back of a book, between the front teeth to save the fingers on the back teeth. Or the assistant may place his thumbs upon the back teeth and push the jaw downward and backward, while he elevates the chin with his fingers, the same care being observed about the sudden closure of the teeth, which always occurs with a snap and great power when the jaw slides into its place. Enveloping the thumbs with several thicknesses of a napkin serves as an additional protection and allows greater pressure to be made. After the jaw has once been dislocated, the accident is liable to occur again; so it should be held while yawning, and while having dental operations performed.

ANÆSTHESIA.

THIS word is applied to that condition in which there is a loss of sensation either in a part or the whole of the body. Any agent that is used to produce that state is called an anæsthetic; the latter word is also used as an adjective to designate the class. Chloroform, ether, nitrous oxide, bichloride of methylene, etc., are agents used to produce general anæsthesia. Of these chloroform, ether, or a mixture of the two, are most commonly used for extensive surgical operations; although occasionally used in the extraction of teeth, they are so seldom employed that it will be an unnecessary consumption of space to treat of them particularly.

Nitrous oxide is, *par excellence*, applicable to the extraction of teeth, on account of the speedy production and the short duration of the anæsthetic state produced by it. A separate chapter will be devoted to its consideration.

Various applications also have been made to the parts about the teeth for the production of local anæsthesia, with more or less successful results. Pounded ice and salt contained in a small bag and held in contact with the teeth and gums until the parts are benumbed; and the production of cold by pumping on a spray of ether or rhigolene, are means that have frequently succeeded well in removing the pain of extraction. Applications of equal parts of chloroform and tincture of aconite root, and of a mixture of camphor and ether, have resulted very satisfactorily in obtunding sensibility. It must be recollected that the tincture of aconite is very poisonous, and should be used with great care.

Another method which has probably been more successful than any other, with the exception of general anæsthesia, consists in the passage of an electric current through the tooth at the time of extraction. Any one who has felt the "shock" of an ordinary electro-galvanic battery, can appreciate how that sensation might overcome the pain of tooth-drawing. Occasionally persons are found, however, that object to the "needles and pins" feeling so much, that they would rather suffer the pain of extraction.

The advantage of these agents for producing local anæsthesia, is that they are safe, without regard to age, sex, or conditions of the mind or body. Objections to the use of the ether spray have been made on the ground that intense cold sometimes causes sloughing of the gums I do not recognize any danger from this unless the application should be prolonged to an unnecessary extent. Dr. Garretson, than whom there is probably no better authority in matters connected with surgery, says: "An objection urged to the use of extreme cold as thus induced, is, that injury is done to the soft parts, as it is thought will be manifested in inability to unite wounds happily and easily. That such objection is, however, not valid, I have satisfactorily proven, for, if any thing, parts thus operated on have united better and with less inflammatory reaction than has obtained where the spray has not been used." There is no circumstance in life which exhibits in a more marked manner the differences between people than the varying degrees of ability or willingness to bear the extraction of teeth. A small and sickly person, on the one hand, may laugh at the idea of any body not having manhood or womanhood enough to bear it, while on the other, a person almost giant-like in strength and stature may faint at the thoughts of the operation and suffer for years all the ills arising from diseased teeth, rather than submit to it. Others again, and not a few, think it sinful to tamper with human life by taking anæsthetics for such a trivial operation as the extraction of teeth.

NITROUS OXIDE GAS.

NITROUS OXIDE, Protoxide of Nitrogen or "Laughing Gas," was discovered in 1776 by the celebrated English chemist, Dr. Priestley. For more than twenty years it excited very little interest, until Sir Humphrey Davy, in 1799, began his celebrated "Researches."

One volume of his works is almost entirely devoted to his investigations, and in one of his note-books kept at the time is the following allusion to them: "These experiments have been made since April, 1799, the period when I first breathed nitrous oxide. Ten months of incessant labor were employed in making them, three months in detailing them." This gas, composed of nitrogen and oxygen, one equivalent of each, is but one of the many instances of the wonders of chemical combination as compared with mechanical mixture. A measure of salt or sugar mixed with one, two, three or more measures of water, makes only a compound more or less salt or sweet, without affecting its nature; but in chemical combination, a measure more or less makes the difference between a solid and a fluid, or a gas—an inert substance, or a deadly poison.

Thus, *five* equivalents of oxygen and *one* of nitrogen give us nitric acid, or aqua fortis, an intensely sour, colorless and powerfully corrosive liquid; *four* equivalents of oxygen and *one* of nitrogen form hyponitric acid, an orange-colored liquid with cherry-red vapor, boiling at 82° and solidifying at 8°; *three* of oxygen and *one* of nitrogen yield nitrous acid, an orange-red vapor, a poor supporter of combustion and very destructive to life; *two* of oxygen and *one* of nitrogen form nitric oxide, or deutoxide of nitrogen, a colorless gas that extinguishes burning substances and is fatal to animal life; *one* equivalent of nitrogen and *one* of oxygen furnish us with nitrous oxide, the subject of our study; while a mechanical mixture of four parts nitrogen and one of oxygen, constitutes the air we breathe.

Nitrous oxide is a colorless gas of sweetish odor and taste, heavier than the air, almost as vigorous a supporter of combustion as pure oxygen, and can be breathed not only without injury in the vast majority of cases, but often with real benefit.

To make it, nitrate of ammonia is placed in a retort and exposed to the heat of a flame, which decomposes it into water and nitrous oxide; the latter passing through the wash-jars and being collected in the gasometer. Nitrate of ammonia is the salt produced by the combination of nitric acid and ammonia. Nitric acid, we have seen, is composed of nitrogen and oxygen; and ammonia is formed of hydrogen and nitrogen. By decomposing at the proper heat, the elements choose to combine in another manner; some of the oxygen uniting with hydrogen to form water, and the rest with nitrogen to form the gas. Great care is required in keeping the heat at the proper point during the generation of the gas, as a temperature a little too high causes the formation of poisonous vapors.

It is a responsibility that few dentists ought to take upon themselves, especially since the invention, by Mr. Sprague, of Boston, of an attachment which automatically regulates the heat upon principles philosophically certain. Then the nitrate of ammonia should be perfectly pure, and a series of wash-bottles interposed between the retort and the gasometer, should contain the requisite purifying chemicals to arrest the slight impurities that arise, no matter how carefully the operation is conducted. The gas should then stand over water from eight to ten hours, —or a day or two would even be better. "Fresh gas every day," sounds well to those who associate freshness with excellence, but some things are better for being a little old. Epicures would hardly patronize the vender who advertised fresh whisky, fresh wines, fresh cigars, fresh pickles, fresh cheese, etc. But operators that administer the gas much, have not time to let it stand, so people that object to old gas need not be afraid of getting it. Although absolute freshness is *not* an advantage, absolute purity *is;* and the way to secure pure gas is to have the best apparatus, the purest chemicals, sufficient chemical knowledge and careful manipulation.

The gas should be inhaled through a mouth-piece which has the valves arranged so that what is expired from the lungs can not re-enter the vessel containing the gas. This method is far superior to the old one of breathing from and into a rubber bag, the contents of which became more and more poisoned with carbonic acid from the patient's lungs at each succeeding breath. In that way the person was often as much smothered by the carbonic acid, as influenced by the nitrous oxide; but because consciousness of pain was lost, the end was supposed to be gained. So it could have been gained about as well by lowering the patient into the choke-damp of a well, until unconsciousness was produced.

Before inhaling the gas, the mind should be free from all fear either in regard to the possibility of pain or of dangerous consequences from the inhalation; not that the imagination of evil effects will cause them to occur, but it may make a very unpleasant and disagreeable operation of what otherwise would be a delightful one.

There should be a perfect willingness or even anxiety to inhale it, and the thoughts should be fixed as much as possible upon some pleasing subject, such as music, scenery, travel, etc. In nine out of ten of those cases where persons fail to become perfectly unconscious, or where they express themselves as being disagreeably affected, the cause is to be found in some dread or fear that impressed itself firmly in the mind at the outset. One common cause, especially with ladies, is the determination not to say anything while under the influence that may cause them embarrassment. Such anxiety I believe to be perfectly unjustifiable, for in daily administrations of the gas for six years, I never had a patient make use of an indelicate remark, or do or say anything that would cause regret. It is very rare indeed that a person who takes nitrous oxide for the purpose of having teeth extracted, says a word. It is not as it is in its administration at humorous exhibitions, for then the gas is taken away just as soon as the period of excitement is reached; those who dance, sing, laugh, fight, speak, etc., would keep perfectly quiet and pass into the anæsthetic state, just as in having teeth extracted, if not prevented.

The power of studied resolves to interfere with the usual effects of anæsthetic agents has long been known. Bouisson gives the case of a young soldier that feigned disease to avoid military service; he was placed under the influence of ether, it being supposed that his answers to questions would betray him, but "he played his part so well as a dissimulator, as never to respond to any question in such a way as to compromise himself." In detailing the effects of an administration of ether to himself, M. Gerdy says: "My lids seemed heavy. I wished to sleep, and above all to abandon myself to the charm which intoxicated me; nevertheless, because *I wished absolutely to observe myself to the last moment*, I did not abandon myself to the seduction which was fascinating me, and I did not sleep. I remarked immediately, that with the exception of certain vibratory sensations which generalized my sense of touch and blunted the sense of pain, and with the exception of a roaring in my ears which prevented my clearly distinguishing what I heard, my perceptions and my thoughts were very clear and my intelligence perfectly free." In the majority of cases, the gas is taken with pleasant feelings, the anæsthesia is produced without trouble, several teeth are extracted without the patient's knowledge or resistance, and on awaking the operation is declared pleasant, or at least not disagreeable. About a minute may be considered the average time for producing the anæsthetic state, and its continuance may be estimated at three-quarters of a minute. But sometimes persons are met with who take longer to get under the influence and remain anæsthetized for a greater time; others declare that they knew everything that was going on, but felt no pain and could not resist. Others knew nothing nor felt nothing, but the general sensation was very disagreeable; and occasionally individuals are met with who appear not to be affected by the gas at all, even after breathing large quantities of it.

The sensations existing during the operation, are expressed in various ways, and it seems in fact that no two persons are affected in all respects exactly alike, with the exception of those who have no recollection at all of their impressions. It may not be uninteresting to give a few instances of remarkable variations from the usual experience had in the administration. A young lady, accompanied by her father, came into the office to have an upper molar extracted. She inhaled the gas properly, but just as the mouthpiece was removed, she closed her teeth firmly together and held them so until she opened her eyes and began, apparently, to awake. She had consumed the contents of the gasometer, so her father told her to have it pulled without gas. She obediently opened her mouth and turned her head far around for the light to fall upon the tooth, which was then extracted; but in reply to our inquiries, she informed us that she did not know when the tooth was extracted, and had nothing but most pleasant sensations.

In another case, a young lady who had inhaled the gas at several offices without being put to sleep, as she said, wished to have a couple of badly decayed front teeth extracted. She inhaled two or three times the amount of gas usually required, and kept shaking her head negatively during the whole time, to signify that she was not under the influence. I took the inhaler from her mouth and she at once began to cry out and to repeat: "Don't you dare to pull my teeth; I am just as conscious as you are!" In accordance with the directions of her elder sister, however, who previously told me to extract them in any manner that was possible, I proceeded to apply the forceps, regardless of her remonstrances, and succeeded in removing the teeth. We were greatly surprised afterward to find that she possessed no recollection of what had occurred. She probably had been in the same peculiar condition at the other dental offices, but they did not feel justified in pulling her teeth, which I certainly would not have done, if I had not received the instructions I did from her sister.

Another case was that of a girl of very nervous temperament. While the preparations were being made to administer the gas, she fainted through fright. I extracted her teeth while she was thus unconscious and then brought her to by sprinkling water on her face and arms. She appeared to know that she had fainted, but not knowing of her teeth being drawn, she began to prepare herself to inhale the gas.

Another case is that of a gentleman, who came into the office to have some filling done. Seeing the gasometer and the inhaling tube before him, he requested a breath or two of the gas, observing at the same time that he had a carious wisdom-tooth that he wished extracted some day, but wanted to see somebody inhale the gas before he ventured to take it to the point of unconsciousness. He took only two or three breaths, when he let the inhaler slip from his mouth. Seeing that he was in the anæsthetic state, I seized the opportunity and extracted his tooth. Almost immediately he came to, expressing his belief that it would be impossible to anæsthetize him. It is needless to depict his astonishment when the tooth was shown him. The sight of blood was insufficient to convince him, mirrors and touch having to be employed in addition.

All things considered, I have certainly had by far the happiest results when nitrous oxide has been administered to people of intellectual culture, who have read or heard of the delightful experience of others of the same class, and who possessing poetical imaginations, or longings to partake of the same spiritual feasts, are anxious to enter the dreamy, blissful state that generally follows the inhalation of *pure* gas, when the mind is untrammeled with dread or fear.

People of the grosser kinds without refinement or mental culture, and those without any appreciation of the exalting influences of this exhilarating agent, may be either pleasantly or unpleasantly affected as it happens; just as a man may get drunk and enjoy it, or get drunk and be sick. What certainty is there in pleasant results from the administration of nitrous oxide to rough, ignorant persons that call for "gas" which they know by no other name, and wonder that it comes from a special gasometer, instead of the tube for illuminating gas; or want to know, when water is handed them in a glass, if that's "the stuff?"

I have in mind a case connected with just such an individual. He couldn't or wouldn't understand; he wouldn't keep his lips tightly closed around the mouth-piece; he either breathed as quick and short as a worried cat, or with the labor of an asthmatic patient; he persisted in keeping his eyes open; he said the gas was sweet or not, pleasant or not, just as he imagined you wanted him to.

Finally he got his eyes shut and refused to answer questions. My patience gave out, and I concluded that his habitual lack of sensibility was anæsthesia enough for him; so I told him he was asleep now and asked him if I should pull his teeth. He gave his consent, and I wrenched out a large molar; he wanted to spit, but as I feared he would pass out of the anæsthetic state, I told him to hold on till I got the other two out. He stood it manfully, and when I got through he jumped up, slapped me on the back and said: "Gas iss the best ding—I never have him pull no oder vay." He had not inhaled a particle of the gas, but was immensely satisfied, and I don't know how many patients his recommendation brought me.

In order to acquaint those who have not had their attention called to the subject, with some of the effects of nitrous oxide, I will give some extracts from the recorded evidence of Sir Humphrey Davy, and others who lent him their aid in his researches:

"The first inspirations occasioned a slight degree of giddiness, succeeded by a sensation analogous to gentle pressure on all the muscles, attended by a highly pleasurable thrilling, particularly in the chest and the extremities. The objects around me became dazzling, and my hearing more acute. Toward the last inspirations, the thrilling increased, the sense of muscular power became greater, and at last an irresistible propensity to action was indulged in: I recollect but indistinctly what followed; I know that my motions were various and violent."

"By degrees, as the pleasurable sensations increased, I lost all connection with external things; trains of vivid visible images rapidly passed through my mind, and were connected with words in such a manner, as to produce perceptions perfectly novel. I existed in a world of newly connected and newly modified ideas. I theorized—I imagined that I made discoveries. When I was awakened from this semi-delirious trance by Dr. Kingslake, who took the bag from my mouth, indignation and pride were the first feelings produced by the sight of the persons around me. My emotions were enthusiastic and sublime; and for a minute I walked round the room, perfectly regardless of what was said to me. As I recovered my former state of mind, I felt an inclination to communicate the discoveries I had made during the experiment. I endeavored to recall the ideas, they were feeble and indistinct; one collection of terms, however, presented itself; and with the most intense belief and prophetic manner, I exclaimed to Dr. Kingslake, 'Nothing exists but thoughts! the universe is composed of impressions, ideas, pleasures and pains.'"

"On May 5, at night, after walking for an hour amid the scenery of the Avon, at this period rendered exquisitely beautiful by bright moonshine; my mind being in a state of agreeable feeling, I respired six quarts of newly prepared nitrous oxide. The thrilling was very rapidly produced. * * * The pleasurable sensation was at first local, and perceived in the lips and about the cheeks. It gradually, however, diffused itself over the whole body, and in the middle of the experiment was for a moment so intense and pure as to absorb existence. At this moment, and not before, I lost consciousness. * * * The thrilling and the pleasurable feeling continued for many minutes; I felt, two hours afterward, a slight recurrence of them in the intermediate state between sleeping and waking, and I had during the whole of the night vivid and agreeable dreams."

"Of two paralytic patients who were asked what they felt after breathing nitrous oxide, the first answered: 'I do not know how, but very queer.' The second said: 'I felt like the sound of a harp.'"

The above extracts are taken from several of Sir Humphrey Davy's experiments. His friend, Mr. Tobin, thus expressed himself after inhalation of the gas:

"It is not easy to describe my sensations; they were superior to anything I ever before experienced. My step was firm, and all my muscular powers increased. My senses were more alive to every surrounding impression; I threw myself into several theatrical attitudes, and traversed the laboratory with a quick step; my mind was elevated to a most sublime height. It is giving but a faint idea of the feelings to say that they resembled those produced by a representation of an heroic scene on the stage, or by reading a sublime passage in poetry, when circumstances contribute to awaken the finest sympathies of the soul. In a few minutes the usual state of mind returned. I continued in good spirits for the rest of the day and slept soundly."

Mr. Wm. Clayfield said: "I was for some time unconscious of existence, but at no period of the experiment experienced agreeable sensations; a momentary nausea followed it, but unconnected with languor or headache."

The poet, Southey, thus expressed himself: "In breathing the nitrous oxide, I could not distinguish between the first feelings it occasioned and an apprehension of which I was unable to divest myself. My first definite sensation was a dizziness, a fullness in the head, such as to induce a fear of falling. This was momentary. When I took the bag from my mouth, I immediately laughed. The laugh was involuntary but highly pleasurable, accompanied by a thrill all through me, and a tingling in my toes and fingers, a sensation perfectly new and delightful. I felt a fullness in my chest afterward; and during the remainder of the day, imagined that my taste and hearing were more than commonly quick. Certain I am that I felt myself more than usually strong and cheerful. * * * Now after an interval of some months, during which my health has been materially impaired, the nitrous oxide produces an effect upon me totally different. Half the quantity affects me, and its operation is more violent, a slight laughter is first induced, and a desire to continue the inhalation, which is counteracted by fear from the rapidity of respiration; indeed, my breath becomes so short and quick, that I have no doubt that the quantity which I formerly breathed would now destroy me. The sensation is not painful, neither is it in the slightest degree pleasurable."

[After this letter was written, he again had pleasant effects.]

Coleridge, the poet, said: "My sensations were highly pleasurable, not so intense or apparently local, but of more unmingled pleasure than I had ever before experienced."

Mr. Wansey thus expressed himself: "The effect was gradual, and I at first experienced fullness of the head, and afterward sensations so delightful that I can compare them to no others, except those which I felt (being a lover of music) about five years since in Westminster Abbey, in some of the grand choruses in the Messiah, from the united power of seven hundred instruments."

Mr. Coates wrote in a letter to Mr. Davy: "During the rest of the day, I experienced a degree of hilarity altogether new to me. For six or seven days afterward, I seemed to feel most exquisitely at every nerve, and was much indisposed to my sedentary pursuits; this acute sensibility has been gradually diminishing; but I still feel somewhat of the effects of this novel agent."

"Joseph Priestley, from breathing nitrous oxide, generally had unpleasant fullness of the head and throbbing of the arteries, which prevented him from continuing the respiration."

R. Boulton and G. Watt were less affected than any. These quotations are enough to show what pleasurable feelings generally attend the inhalation of nitrous oxide; by them we see also that people were affected in different ways and degrees, then as well as now. The gas being inhaled from a bag, if it had been taken to the state of profound anæsthesia often, as it is now, unpleasant sensations would have been more frequent, on account of the complete exhaustion of the nitrous oxide and the substitution of carbonic acid from the lungs.

Certain it is that with the improved facilities of recent times, safety and pleasure ought to exist to even a greater degree. If they do not, it must be attributable to the fact that in those days there was no previous unsettling of the mind by the suffering of toothache and the dread of extraction. Those who inhale the gas for curiosity alone nowadays, seem to experience even greater pleasure than experimenters did in the time of Davy. I know that in my own case language is too tame to describe the brilliant conceptions, bright visions and glorious imagery that fill my mind at those times when every external influence is removed and my soul appears to float away through space; although I imagine while in that state that it will be my pleasure and duty to communicate my thoughts, and that I shall be able to do so without any of that embarrassment that so often mortifies me in speaking.

With Sir Humphrey Davy originated the idea of using nitrous oxide to prevent pain during short surgical operations. Says he: "As nitrous oxide in its extensive operation appears capable of destroying physical pain, it may probably be used with advantage during surgical operations in which no great effusion of blood takes place."

In another place: "The power of the immediate operation of the gas in removing intense physical pain, I had a very good opportunity of ascertaining. In cutting one of the unlucky teeth called *dentes sapientiæ*, I experienced an extensive inflammation of the gum, accompanied with great pain, which equally destroyed the power of repose, and of consistent action. On the day when the inflammation was most troublesome, I breathed three large doses of nitrous oxide. The pain always diminished after the first four or five inspirations; the thrilling came on as usual, and uneasiness was for a few minutes swallowed up in pleasure." It would be impossible for any man to have such thoughts, without having at once forced upon his mind the idea of the painless extraction of teeth by the use of nitrous oxide. If Sir Humphrey Davy or any one of the friends that experimented with him had been a *dentist*, there is no doubt that it would have been so applied at once; but when we consider that dentistry was almost unknown and that the manufacture of gas in its purity was difficult and the knowledge confined to practical chemists, it is not be wondered at that its application for dental purposes was deferred until a recent period. The advantageous use of nitrous oxide for certain bodily complaints began to be noticed at the same time. For the later investigations concerning its medical uses in asthma, consumption and other diseases, the reader is referred to an excellent work on Nitrous Oxide, by Dr. George J. Ziegler, of Philadelphia.

No matter what ignorance may exist in regard to the gas and its physiological effects, there are very few that doubt its power to speedily and certainly place them in such a condition that operations may be painlessly performed; but a vast number of people have serious doubts as to its safety, and the question is constantly heard, "Is it dangerous to take the gas?" The correctness of the answer "No," depends upon the conception of the meaning of "dangerous." My opinion is that the only true way of answering the question to each one's satisfaction is by comparing the number of accidents resulting from the inhalation of gas with those resulting from a thousand and one other things that people are constantly doing, and yet do not consider them especially "dangerous."

Let a hundred thousand people go carriage-riding, go gunning, cross the Atlantic, take a long railroad journey, or take medicine, and far more fatality would result than if the same people inhaled nitrous oxide to unconsciousness. Yet people are constantly doing these things voluntarily and gladly, and when fatal accidents occur no one is blamed and the survivors straightway do the same things again. But if one death should occur in twice a hundred thousand administrations of nitrous oxide, I doubt not that the public would become greatly alarmed and gas would grow stale in the gasometer, unless the dentist should happen to have a grain of confidence left and use it up himself for fun.

The subjoined statistical report, based upon the impartial examination of a number of cases by Prof. E. Andrews, and published in the Chicago Medical Examiner, speaks a volume in favor of the safety of nitrous oxide compared with other anæsthetics:

Ether,	1 death to	23.204	administrations.
Chloroform,	1 " "	2.723	"
Mixed Chloroform and Ether,	1 " "	5.588	"
Bichloride of Methylene,	1 " "	7.000	"
Nitrous Oxide,	No " "	75.000	"

Mr. Sprague, of Boston, well known in connection with nitrous oxide and the improved apparatus for generating it, reports that he has taken the gas to insensibility "nearly two hundred times within the last three years, with beneficial rather than injurious results." There have been only three or four fatal cases that have been attributed to the use of nitrous oxide, and those have been attended with extenuating circumstances. One was that of a gentleman in New

York, nearly dead of consumption, who died a few hours afterward. Another was that of a young lady of Vermont, suffering with a disease of the membranes of the brain and spinal cord, who died several days after inhaling the gas for amusement. Another case was that of a gentleman who died in Philadelphia before leaving the dental office, and whose death was supposed to result from a tooth or piece of cork, that was known to have entered his windpipe. Some four years ago, a woman died on the street not long after inhaling the gas at some office in Cincinnati; but the Coroner attributed her death to another cause altogether. Numerous reports have been made, however, of serious and enduring systemic injury resulting from notably impure gas, or even from purer gas indiscreetly administered without regard to certain mental and bodily conditions. From all the evidence that has been adduced, it may be argued that pure nitrous oxide, administered with discretion in proper cases, is *safe*. Such administrations as that noticed in Sprague's treatise, are *hardly* safe. "At this time, a lady acquaintance in delicate health applied to one of those 'Pure Gas' offices, to have an offending molar removed by gas. While she waited, a furious heat was applied to a pint retort charged with a crude salt, and the gas forced rapidly through a single small washing-bottle into a four-gallon bag. Soon the bloated bag was brought out, the lady gagged with a cork, the mouth-piece forced between her jaws, and she left, *nolens volens*, to breathe this compound of corruption. Insensibility *from some cause* soon followed, and the tooth was drawn. Upon recovering consciousness, she experienced a violent headache, nausea, and a sore mouth. The irritation of her lungs was also increased, and for weeks she was a severe sufferer. Her experience assured her, and the whole community, that nitrous oxide was not safe. Friends and neighbors, and 'all the doctors' of the village, joined in condemning the use of such a dangerous agent as nitrous oxide, while not a suspicion rested upon the knowledge and skill of the 'excellent dentist.' "

In regard to the poisonous vapors that may be formed by fluctuations of heat, Prof. Geo. Watt says: "No man can give such attention to the process, with ordinary apparatus, as will enable him to *know* that he has not a mixture of nitrous and nitric oxyds in his gasometer instead of *pure nitrous oxyd*. With the uncertainty of the ordinary processes of decomposing nitrate of ammonia it is not strange that congestion and soreness of the air-passages are so frequently observed after the use of the nitrous oxyd. Defective apparatus in the hands of the inexperienced, and those without chemical education, is likely to result imperfectly. * * * Though a teacher of chemistry for nearly a quarter of a century, I never would, *never did*, and NEVER WILL use a nitrous oxyd apparatus, even for amusement, without the ability absolutely to control the temperature at which the gas is generated."

But even where the gas is perfectly pure there should much judgment be used before its administration is decided upon. In cases where the increased force of the circulation, arising from its use, *might* be of serious disadvantage, great caution should always be observed, and sometimes it should not be administered at all.

It is not good policy to give it in bad cases of heart disease or far advanced pulmonary consumption, or to very old people. Such persons are liable to leave the world any day, and if death should happen not long after the inhalation, there would be a distressing state of doubt, as to the cause, existing in both the minds of the patient's friends and the dentist. It is well known that "the pattern of body which is *most* prone to apoplexy is denoted by a large head and red face, shortness and thickness of the neck, and a short, stout, squat build." Great care should be used in giving the gas to such persons, especially after excitement, exercise or full meals; and if they have had any of the premonitory symptoms of apoplexy, or previous attacks, it should *never* be administered. Various temporary derangements of the body, and certain periodical and other conditions of females, should be made the subjects of consultation in order to insure against results of a more or less unpleasant nature. One of the greatest superiorities that nitrous oxide has over ether and chloroform, is in the rapidity with which the patient arouses from its influence upon the admission of air into the lungs, if dangerous symptoms present themselves. There is no cumulative action to render the anæsthetic state more profound after the agent is withdrawn. Were it otherwise, fatal accidents would frequently occur, for nitrous oxide possesses the power of destroying life in a short time, if its inhalation should be continued much too long. But this should be the occasion of no alarm, for there is no more danger of inhaling the gas to that point, than there is of making anything in common use a means of death. A person may drown himself in a basin of water if he will hold his head under long enough. A cat confined in pure nitrous oxide gives up its "nine lives" in three or four minutes. A mouse dies in about a minute. Dr. J. J. Colton, of Philadelphia, says in a treatise recently published: "Man, judging from the appearance of persons in the third stage of anæsthesia, which is effected in from thirty seconds to two minutes, could not survive its inhalation for a longer period than from three to five minutes, depending upon the age, condition of health and susceptibilities to anæsthesia."

In conclusion, I would ask pardon if I have extended my remarks on nitrous oxide to a tiresome degree; but the subject is one of peculiar interest and one upon which the public generally needs information, more than upon any other subject connected with dentistry. Consider what has been said and then " look here upon this picture, and on *this*." An educated dentist, after spending much money and years of time and labor in acquiring knowledge of the subjects connected with his profession, feelingly responds to the entreaties of suffering humanity to save them from pain; regardless of expense, he procures the best apparatus in the market and supplies himself with the purest material; with sleepless eyes he sits hour after hour at night watching his retort and seeing that the slowly bubbling gas on its way to the gasometer through purifying chemicals, carries with it no poisonous vapors. Then when the morning comes and brings his suffering brother to his door, he gives him to drink of this delightful fount from which poets quaff inspiration; leads him with tender hand and watchful care nearly to the "valley of the shadow of death;" relieves him of his suffering, and carefully conducts him back to happy consciousness; and then for all these valuable services, the *grateful* patient thinks, because some uneducated quack has so advertised, that a sufficient remuneration is "FIFTY CENTS." Do not the bones of Priestley, Davy and Wells upheave in indignation the sod that lies over their graves?

DENTIFRICES, BRUSHES, ETC.

MANY people who profess to be very careful of their teeth, do them more harm than good by using injurious preparations. Some depend altogether upon soap as a dentifrice. While it is doubtless useful to destroy the animalcules of the mouth and to facilitate the removal of tenacious mucus, it is generally conceded that its frequent use is injurious to the gums on account of its alkalinity. It does not answer the purpose of a powder nor does a powder that of a soap. It should be used occasionally, care being taken to rinse the mouth thoroughly afterward. Nothing but the purest Castile, or the best cocoa-nut oil soap should be employed.

Charcoal, as usually applied, is very injurious. Many persons are attracted by the readiness with which it removes the stains upon the teeth, and use it freely in its simple pulverized state and combined in the form of paste. Its gritty, insoluble particles insinuate themselves between the teeth and the gums and destroy their connection, frequently producing inflammation of the gums and of the peridental membrane. The finer the charcoal is pulverized the worse it is.

Pumice stone may be spoken of in the same way. The injury arising from these substances may be considered hardly appreciable, where they are employed only occasionally and applied with a pointed stick, care being taken not to lodge them under the gums, and to rinse the mouth thoroughly. Nothing is better in the way of a simple grit than cigar ashes; it does its work well and is soluble. One of the best tooth powders for general use is the following:

"Precipitated carbonate of lime, . . . 4 ounces.
Pulverized orris root, ... $\frac{3}{4}$ ounce.
" white sugar, ... 1$\frac{1}{4}$ ounce.
" slippery elm bark, . . . $\frac{1}{4}$ ounce.
" cuttle-fish bone, . . . $\frac{1}{4}$ ounce."

Color with carmine and flavor with oil of wintergreen or rose. Persons making the powder for themselves, should be provided with a mortar and pestle with which to incorporate the ingredients, and a very fine sieve to rub the powder through when finished.

In coloring, the carmine and cuttle-fish bone are first ground together, and the other ingredients then added.

Another is made thus:

"Precipitated carbonate of lime, . . . 4 ounces.
Pulverized orris root, ... 2 ounces.
Prepared oyster shell, ... 2 ounces."
Color and flavor if desirable.

A good and very simple powder is made by mixing equal parts of prepared chalk and powdered orris root, and adding a little of the scrapings of fine soap.

These powders are all that are necessary where the teeth and mouth are in a healthy condition; if tartar or diseased gums exist, the dentist should be consulted. The objects of the use of the powders are to counteract acidity of the mouth, and to *prevent* the accumulation of tartar after the teeth have been cleaned. It can be laid down as a rule that any advertised preparation that whitens the teeth speedily, is injurious to the substance of the teeth, and, in fact, it is unsafe to resort to them anyhow. The dentist can furnish preparations that will do all the good possible, and at the same be harmless, although he may not get them up in such handsome bottles or boxes, nor with such pretentious labels.

A good and pleasant mouth wash, in cases of fetid breath, inflamed gums, etc., is made thus.

Tincture of krameria,	3 fluid ounces.
Eau de Cologne,	6 fluid ounces
Oil of wintergreen,	10 drops.

Of this mixture add a teaspoonful or two to a wine-glass of water.

The best brushes are those which have the bristles pointed instead of being cut with square ends; they enter between the teeth better. The stiffness of the bristles must depend upon the condition of the gums. If they bleed easily, a soft brush must be first used, but perfectly healthy gums ought to bear without injury the stiffest brush.

The proper method of cleaning the teeth is particularly noticed in the chapter on Prevention of Caries.

TOBACCO.

THOSE who are addicted to the habits of smoking and chewing to excess, generally attribute to them whatever bad teeth they may have, and are continually asking the dentist, "Is tobacco injurious to the teeth?" Not that an answer confirming their suspicion would cause them to free themselves from their bondage, but they appear curious to know the full extent of their sufferings from their self-inflicted martyrdom.

I believe that the *direct* effect of tobacco upon the substance of the teeth is not injurious—possibly slightly beneficial from its pain allaying and saliva increasing properties; but this is no argument in favor of its use, for when used to any great extent, its *indirect* evil effects are too evident. Whatever lessens the nutrition, health and vigor of the system, injures the parts associated intimately with the teeth, their susceptibility to certain diseases being increased and their recuperative power decreased. Anything that deranges the digestive organs, and causes acidity of the stomach and sour regurgitations, produces a condition very unfavorable to the preservation of the teeth. These, tobacco is certainly capable of doing, and besides, it is a notorious fact, that the greater slaves people become to tobacco, the more uncleanly do they become in regard to their teeth. Many dentists give it as their experience, that a larger proportion of cases of periodontitis, abscess, abrasion and recession, occur in tobacco users than others, and that they are less amenable to treatment. That severe constitutional disorders should follow the unrestrained use of such a powerful agent as tobacco, can not be wondered at when we consider the virulence of its poisonous principle, and the number of its poisonous adulterations. A single drop of this principle, nicotin, will kill a good-sized dog, and birds die at the approach, only, of a vial containing it. Antimony, lead, copper, copperas, corrosive sublimate, etc., are some of the adulterations. Indigestion, emaciation, neuralgia, paralysis, insanity, heart disease, and a disorder much like delirium tremens, have been ascribed to the abuse of tobacco.

In France, of late years, a commission was "appointed to inquire into the influence of tobacco in the schools and colleges." It was ascertained that those who did not use it were so much better physically, morally and intellectually, that "an edict was issued, prohibiting the use of tobacco in these national institutions, by which thirty thousand persons were at once forced to abandon it."

Dr. Willard Parker, of New York, says: "Cigar-makers, snuff manufacturers, etc., have come under my care in hospitals and in private practice, and such persons *never* recover soon and in a healthy manner, from any case of injury or fever. They are more apt to die in epidemics, and are more prone to apoplexy and paralysis. The same is true also, of all who *chew and smoke much.*" Bearing these facts in mind, it is easy to believe that diseases about the mouths of tobacco-chewers are more violent and less easily cured, than those of other persons.

It would of course be vain to expect that the devotees of tobacco would sacrifice the habit that enthralls them, for the sake of their *teeth*, when the most powerful arguments that are prompted by the fear of mental and bodily diseases fail to break the spell; but it may not be unreasonable to hope that a compromise may be effected by which the pleasures of the habit will not be detracted from, and yet the injurious effects will be lessened, and the demands of cleanliness and decency better answered. After every smoke or chew, brush the teeth thoroughly, rinse the mouth and gargle the throat; thus the absorption of much poison, and the waste of much saliva will be prevented. Afterward, especially before going into society, use some fragrant tooth-powder, and I promise you that your teeth will be better preserved, and you will cease to be disgusting to your friends that are not tobacco users. No person of refinement, whether patient or dentist, should give or receive the offense of a breath impregnated with the odor of tobacco, which is always disagreeable in close quarters. Many that find it beyond their power to give up tobacco entirely find very little trouble in reducing the number of "chews" or "smokes," and the quantity used each time. The more saliva saved, and the less poison of tobacco and adulterations absorbed, the better for health and teeth.

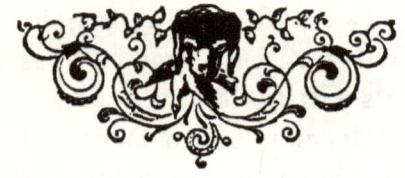

ARTIFICIAL TEETH.

AFTER the loss of a few or all of the teeth by negligence, accident or disease, it becomes the duty of the dentist to insert artificial substitutes.

Such has been the advancement of this art during the last few years that now any number of teeth from one to a full set can be inserted, and in the majority of cases can be made to resemble the natural teeth so nearly in appearance and usefulness, that the loss is scarcely felt. Considering how essential the teeth are to good looks, mastication, enunciation, good health and enjoyment of life, it is fortunate that the dentist possesses such skill. Yet it is to be lamented that so many thousands of people appreciate the natural teeth so slightly, that they suffer them to go by default and would rather have artificial teeth than submit to some inconvenience and a little more expense in preserving those that nature gave them. Such a course is certainly a violation of natural laws and doubtless brings its punishment, for I believe it to be a fact that the average duration of life in those that lose their teeth early and resort to artificial ones, is not so great as in those that preserve their own teeth to late in life. But after the natural teeth are lost, of course the health is improved and life prolonged to a greater extent by having artificial substitutes, than by going without them.

There is no branch of dentistry that requires more skill and general knowledge than the *proper* insertion of artificial teeth. The plates should fit the mouth well and be so applied as to exert no injurious influence upon the soft parts or upon the natural teeth, if any should remain. The articulation of the teeth should imitate nature as nearly as possible,—the cusps and prominences of one set being received into the depressions of the other so as to secure perfect antagonism and occlusion; this is so important for mastication and enunciation. They should not be cumbersome on account of their bulk, while they should be of sufficient strength to withstand all legitimate usage. The color should be suitable for the age, sex and complexion of the patient, or should correspond perfectly with remaining natural teeth.

The size and shape should be appropriate for each individual case. The material of which the plates are composed, should be of such recognized purity as to preclude the possibility of injurious local or systemic effects.

The arrangement of the teeth and the perfection of the work should be such that they would not be suspected to be artificial. The teeth and plate should be so accurately joined as to prevent the insinuation of particles of food. The dentist should possess enough of the talent of the portrait artist to restore the natural facial expression ; and, finally, realizing that no two cases are precisely alike, he should be endowed with that versatility which enables the skillful dentist to accommodate all of those little peculiarities that are constantly presenting themselves. There is no doubt that first-class dentists everywhere are fast losing their interest in mechanical dentistry, and the people are to blame for the change. The dentist knows what judgment, skill and labor are required ; but the people, not having a just appreciation, are often unwilling to half pay him for his services, and rush with eagerness to the cheap charlatan, who gives them a mouthful of something to shout his praise and make excuse for their own penuriousness by abusing the extravagant charges of those dentists who can not consistently sacrifice their consciences and the last vestige of their professional dignity by descending to the level of the quack in recommending cheap materials, cheaply put together without regard to the patient's welfare.

From what has been written in the previous pages, it will be understood that the preservation of the natural teeth is to be advised in nearly all cases, in preference to resorting to artificial ones. An exception exists sometimes in the case of deforming, irremediable irregularity. After one or more teeth have been lost, it is nearly always advisable to insert artificial ones, unless the natural teeth are so crowded that the space is of advantage. A natural tooth should not be left without an antagonist, on account of its subsequent elongation and loss. If an artificial tooth should not be needed for appearance or speech, nor particularly for mastication, it is often required to prevent the adjoining teeth from becoming irregular.

PREPARATION OF THE MOUTH.

To secure the best satisfaction from a full or partial set of artificial teeth, care should be taken to put the mouth in a proper condition before inserting them. Deposits of tartar about any remaining teeth should be removed; decayed teeth should be filled; diseased gums should be cured; and all diseased teeth that can not be restored to a healthy condition should be extracted. It is very bad policy to have a plate inserted over old roots, and yet there are numbers of people that insist on having it done, and will go from dentist to dentist that discountenances the idea, until they find one that to humor them is willing to sacrifice his better judgment and convictions of duty.

The pressure of the plate upon the roots produces inflammation of the surrounding membranes and gums; diseased secretions result which injure the sound teeth, taint the breath and affect the general health. Besides, the resistance of the roots prevents that adaptation of the plate to the mucous membrane which is necessary to keep out particles of food, or to make perfect suction.

When a very few, only, of the natural teeth remain, it is often best to have them removed, even if perfectly sound. This is especially the case where only a few of the front teeth remain, for besides the difficulty of so perfectly joining the artificial to the natural gums that they will not be detected, the plate is apt to press away the gums from the necks of the teeth, loosening them and exposing the cementum. This usually involves the trouble and expense of a new plate, for it generally makes a patched job to add new teeth to such plates.

One or two sound molars on each side, can often be left with advantage, especially if they have antagonizing teeth to keep them from being pushed by nature from their sockets.

After the extraction of the teeth, if there are any hanging pieces of gum, they should be cut off. Sharp or projecting portions of bone should be clipped off at the time and the dentist should be called upon occasionally that he may keep them trimmed. If these portions of alveolar process are suffered to remain, they often make the gums very sore, and considerably retard their healing. Tincture of arnica, tincture of calendula, and tincture of myrrh, somewhat diluted, or a decoction of white-oak bark, are excellent for rinsing the mouth to promote the healing of the gums. Rinsing the mouth alternately with warm water and ice-cold water for a number of times as soon as possible after extraction, and afterward using several times a day a wash composed of one-third tincture of arnica and two-thirds water, I have found very successful. It is a good plan to change the washes every few days. The time required for complete healing of the gums of different individuals is quite variable. It depends much upon the number of teeth or roots extracted and their size and firmness in the jaws, the thickness of the alveolar processes, the power of nature to heal wounds in other parts of the body, the attention of the patient, exposure and other circumstances.

TEMPORARY PLATES.

As a general thing it is not advisable to insert temporary sets of artificial teeth; that is those which are usually so-called—teeth without gums, put in within a few days after extraction. The impression of the mouth being taken at that time, the artificial plate has all the irregularities of the alveolar ridge stamped upon it, and besides irritating the tender gums, is apt to prevent them from healing in that smooth and regular manner which is required for a permanent set of teeth, satisfactory in all respects. It is a risk that often has to be run, however, by public speakers, and others who are in such positions that they can not do without their teeth till the mouth is well. Many who have such sets just for appearance sake, are often soon disappointed; for although the teeth may fit accurately into the gums and look naturally at first, the gums in a short time shrink away, leaving a space between them and the teeth.

It is best to wait until the gums have shrunk, at least sufficiently to allow gum-teeth to be inserted without being too prominent; further shrinkage is then not observed, as it is hidden behind the artificial gums, and after it is sure that there will be no further contraction, the same teeth may be taken off and remounted on a new plate. In those cases in which the natural gums are so prominent that, even when entirely healed, they can not have artificial gums placed over them, it is often very hard to tell what course to pursue; if teeth are inserted while any doubts exist as to future contraction, they should be made to press well into the gums, so that a little subsequent shrinkage will not cause a space. But while artificial teeth should not be inserted too soon, on the other hand it is wrong to leave them out too long. Where all the teeth on either or both jaws have been removed, the lips and cheeks are apt to lose their natural expression, and the lower jaw often becomes partially dislocated and inclined to project; the gums, moreover, having become callous by long usage, it is much more difficult to adapt plates to them. If natural teeth are left in either jaw without antagonists, they become much elongated in course of time, sometimes coming so near to the opposite gum that artificial teeth can not be inserted without cutting away a great deal of the natural teeth.

SUCTION AND CLASP PLATES.

Entire sets of artificial teeth used to be kept in the mouth by the constant pressure of springs, extending from the upper to the lower plates; but it was found that often after the breaking of the springs, the lower plate would remain in position by its own weight, and that the upper one would stay on account of the complete exhaustion of air between it and the mucous membrane. From this it was ascertained that the springs might be abandoned altogether by having the upper plates larger and perfectly adapted. Upper plates, either full or partial, are, nowadays, hardly ever inserted any other way. A good fit to the roof of the mouth is generally sufficient, but usually there is an air-chamber in addition carved out of the plate next to the palate, for the purpose of exhausting more air. If suction plates are properly made, much less injury arises from their use than from clasp plates. They should fit the mouth perfectly, the edges of the air-chamber should not injure the palate, the border of the plate, next to the teeth, should not press the gums unduly so as to irritate them, or cause them to recede, and the pressure against the natural teeth should not be so great as to move them much out of their position. Where they are crowded, a slight expansion of the arch is advantageous. Clasp plates have the advantage of small bulk and perfect fixation, but no matter how accurately the clasps may be adapted, they are almost sure in the course of a few years to seriously injure the teeth they are thrown around, if they do not destroy them altogether.

PORCELAIN TEETH.

DENTAL substitutes were formerly made from bone, ivory, human teeth, teeth of cattle, etc.; but of late years these have been entirely superseded by porcelain teeth.

The bulk of the latter is composed chiefly of silex, felspar and a fine variety of white clay, called kaolin; over the surface of the body is melted the enamel, consisting chiefly of felspar. Different substances are added to imitate the various shades of color seen in the teeth and gums; thus oxide of titanium gives yellow; platina sponge and filings, a grayish blue; and oxide of gold, a rose red color. While the teeth are in a soft state, platina pins are sunk into the backs of them and become immovably fixed by subsequent baking at an intense heat.

When well made they are almost perfect imitations of nature, suffer no damage during the process of mounting them on plates, and are unchangeable in the mouth. As with every other article manufactured on so large a scale, the market is flooded with cheap porcelain teeth, poorly made and composed of poor materials.

DIFFERENT KINDS OF PLATES.

It would be quite a task to enumerate the different bases which have been employed from time to time for the purpose of mounting artificial teeth, even without attempting to give a description of them, or to discuss their relative merits. Scarcely a year passes without the discovery of several new bases or methods, which, of course, for the interest of the patentees, must be advertised in the most flattering manner. Some die out about as quickly as they spring into existence, others more slowly, but no less surely; while a few, after a lengthy period of probation, succeed in establishing their claims of excellence. I do not propose to mention particularly any of the bases for artificial teeth, excepting those which are either in general use or have been tested so long that their merits are generally acknowledged; not intending, by so doing, to disparage any of those that are struggling for public recognition, for it is only by such continual experimentation that we can hope to obtain what we never have as yet succeeded in discovering—a base for artificial teeth, perfect in all respects.

CONTINUOUS GUM.

Although but little used, I mention this style of work first, because it surpasses everything else in answering most of the requirements of a perfect set of artificial teeth.

A platina plate is first made to fit the mouth, and then plain teeth, or teeth without gums, are soldered to it. Every portion of the plate, except the surface which is adapted to the mouth, is then coated with a mineral compound like that of which porcelain teeth are made.

Finally, over this coating is melted gum-colored enamel, which joins gums, palate and teeth in one continuous piece without joint or crevice. Both the platina plate and the mineral matter being perfectly pure and unaffected by any agent they may come in contact with, the work is clean, tasteless and durable. As regards its natural appearance, it can be made to defy the closest scrutiny. The teeth can be made to lap over, project, or imitate any little irregularity of the previous natural set; which can not be done with gum teeth mounted on other plates on account of interfering with the jointing of the gums. No matter how much a person may show his gums in laughing or talking, there is no seam shown. The elevation and depression of the natural gums over and between the roots of the teeth, may be perfectly imitated.

Continuous gum work is especially applicable for full upper and lower sets; there are some partial cases in which it can not be used.

The objections urged against it are its weight, liability to fracture, and expensiveness. It certainly weighs much more than any other kind of work, but this is of real advantage in lower sets, and of no disadvantage in upper sets, if the fit is perfect; for if the plate is perfectly adapted to the mucous membrane there is enough atmospheric pressure to sustain many times the weight of the heaviest set of continuous gum teeth.

If it falls on hard places it is more liable to break than other kinds of work, and is more expensive to repair, but it should not be allowed to fall. Fine watches will break in the same way, but I never heard of anybody refusing one on that account. The expensiveness can not be avoided, for the platina is worth nearly as much as gold, and such skill and ingenuity are required that the cheap dentist dares not attempt it.

Mineral plate is but a modification of the above; the platina plate is discarded, and the whole denture is made of the mineral matter. It is superior to the other in lightness, but it can not be made to fit the mouth so well, and it is very liable to fracture.

GOLD PLATES.

For general use, gold plate as a base for artificial teeth, has always held the first place in the estimation of the dentist. It combines great strength with medium weight and slight bulk. It is pure, healthy and unchangeable. One or any number of teeth can be mounted upon it. No matter how often the set may be broken it can be mended again and again without injury to the plate, can be remodeled as often as necessary, and if finally abandoned for another plate, it brings its cash market value. The skillful dentist loves to work with this metal, for he has no better opportunity to show his superiority over the rubber charlatan. In gold plates there is no limit to the display of artistic workmanship, and if the quack ever acquires the necessary skill, he gains such an appreciation of his own labors that he ceases to be a quack.

The objections to gold are these: the fluids of the mouth and portions of food work their way between the teeth and the plate; the teeth are apt to be sprung more or less out of place in the course of time, depending of course much upon the strength of the backings and the power of the masticatory muscles; and the gum of each tooth being ground up to the other, there are a great number of joints made, which are objectionable when persons show their gums. Most of these defects can be remedied by riveting on block teeth, and all of them by attaching block teeth with rubber; but with the exception of the part covering the palate, the set is thereby made about as bulky as a rubber plate.

The expense of gold plates prevents many persons from getting them that prefer them, but where this obstacle can be overcome, a well made gold plate will generally give better satisfaction than anything else, excepting continuous gum.

SILVER PLATES.

A FEW years ago silver was used nearly altogether in those cases where the patient could not afford gold, but since the introduction of rubber, it is fast going into disuse. It makes a strong plate, weighs less than gold, and takes but little room in the mouth. If it would remain as when first put in the mouth, it would still rank next to gold, but it is liable to objectionable changes. The sulphuretted hydrogen of the atmosphere discolors it, as does the sulphur of eggs, mustard, different kinds of game, etc.

It is so acted upon in some mouths, that the plate is corroded through in a few years; occasionally, where kept well cleaned, it is worn for a long time without important change. Silver in its pure state is too soft for dental purposes, and it is generally alloyed with a small portion of copper; many practitioners will not use plate so alloyed, claiming that it often produces serious local and general effects. Platina is the best alloy, preserving the purity of the silver, and remedying the liability to tarnish. Such plates are generally far more durable than the cheaper kinds of work.

CHEOPLASTIC METAL.

THIS is an alloy of tin, silver and bismuth with a small amount of antimony. A trial plate is made upon which to arrange the teeth to suit the case;

this plate is afterward removed from the interior of a flask in which it and the teeth have been incased, and into the vacuum is poured the melted metal. A strong set of teeth is made composed of block or single teeth and a continuous piece of metal holding them in position. The access of fluids and food, and displacement of the teeth are prevented. This is a method but little used, but I have taken it as a representative of several kinds of alloy that are molded into plates in about the same manner. No particular objection is urged against the construction of artificial dentures by such methods, but for some reason or other no one of them has ever been generally adopted, and it is probable it never will. Some of them, however, seem to be preferable to rubber for cheap substitutes.

ALUMINUM PLATES.

Among the many recently introduced bases struggling for precedency, no one presents such auspicious claims as aluminum. It is lighter than any metal used in dentistry, weighing only one-eighth as much as platinum, one-seventh as much as gold, and one-fourth as much as silver. Although it was discovered as long ago as 1827, it is only of late years that it has been produced in sufficient quantities to be of service. Even after the supply became abundant, it was for a long time impossible to either pour a dental plate of it, or to solder teeth to it. Both of the obstacles have been surmounted, and all that aluminum needs to establish its claims of superiority over all of the cheaper bases, is to stand a few years more of trial as successfully as it has done thus far.

It resembles silver somewhat in color, is about as hard, and more tenacious. It neither changes color nor corrodes, and is tasteless. Plain, single gum, or block teeth can be used, and whether the plate is poured, or has the teeth soldered to it, the crevices and joints are filled so as to keep out fluids and food.

"ROSE PEARL."

This romantic name is given to a base of comparatively recent introduction. It is intended as a substitute for continuous gum, and it claims some advantages over that kind of work in that it is by far lighter in weight and much less expensive. The teeth used are single and without gums, so that they can be arranged on a swaged rose-pearl plate, to imitate any irregularity of nature. The material in a plastic state is afterward added to secure the teeth to the plate, and to build out the gums to the required thickness, so that when the work is done, the gums and the plate are united in a continuous piece without any seams showing. The color of the plate, though not a perfect imitation of nature like continuous gum, is tolerably near to it, and much more natural looking than pink rubber.

It has its earnest advocates and its violent opposers. The opposition to it is mainly on the ground that there is so much shrinkage of the material in drying that it is impossible to make a perfect fit. This is doubtless a specious argument, for the added material, spoken of above, is more than half ether, all of which must evaporate, leaving an alveolar border of one-half of the bulk of the original plastic mass. The plate covering the palate, being well seasoned beforehand, may be clamped firmly to the cast while the set is being dried in the oven, but I regard it as simply *impossible* to prevent the parts of the base under the teeth and next to the gums, from drawing away from the cast of the mouth.

Besides, there are always some crevices left about the teeth, which allow the entrance of the fluids of the mouth and fine particles of food. These crevices are only imperfectly closed by pressing down the edges of the material with heated instruments.

Rose-pearl, then, falls short of continuous gum in being not so cleanly, not of such a natural color, and in not being a perfect fit; yet there is no doubt that the perfect adaptation of the plate over the roof of the mouth may be sufficient, in the majority of cases, to retain the plate in position. Some have objected to rose-pearl on account of the taste of its ether in the mouth, and its warping in use. I hardly believe that these things occur, when the plate is thoroughly evaporated before it is inserted. Pyroxyline, a still later base, is, like rose-pearl, a compound of collodion, or gun-cotton. It is open to some of the same objections, while it is not intended to imitate continuous gum at all.

VULCANIZED RUBBER.

For some years rubber has been more commonly used than any other base for artificial teeth. Like everything else it has its merits and its demerits, but, as generally used, the latter certainly outnumber the former.

The best features that it possesses are the perfectness of its adaptation to the mouth, and its cleanliness.

The soft rubber being shaped and hardened upon the original cast of the mouth, a perfect fit is secured: and as all spaces behind and between the teeth are filled up with the base, all fluids and particles of food are excluded. Though not nearly so strong as well made metal plates, it is strong enough for all ordinary purposes; but even this degree of strength can only be secured by a great increase of bulk. Rubber plates, in their thinnest portions, are generally from six to ten times as thick as gold, and in other places from twenty to forty times as thick. Teeth in blocks of three and two generally have to be used, and they can not like single teeth be set in and out to correspond with all the little irregularities of the opposite teeth; as a result, therefore, in the majority of cases, correct articulation is sacrificed for the sake of an evenness, generally unnatural, of the external arch. The joints have to be perfectly made, and care has to be used in pressing the rubber, to prevent the blocks from separating, or cracking, and the rubber from showing.

Rubber plates do not allow frequent repairing as metal plates do; for new rubber having to be added and baked each time, the original plate becomes darker, harder and finally so brittle as to be useless.

They are often much objected to on account of their causing a disagreeable sensation of heat in the mouth; for being such poor conductors, cooling drinks and draughts of air have little effect in lessening the temperature under the plates. From this cause, it is generally conceded that sore, spongy and scalded gums frequently arise. The distressing effects of mercury upon the system have at times been attributed to the use of rubber plates. It has been the subject of much discussion for years, some claiming that mercury as incorporated in the coloring matter of the rubber is inert, and others asserting that it is capable of exercising all of its poisonous properties. The subject of mercurial poisoning has been noticed in the article on Amalgam.

Reputable dentists, everywhere, are opposed to the use of rubber, although they have to employ it to meet the public demand; for it has done much toward detracting from the dignity of the profession and interfering with its advancement. The process of fitting a rubber plate to the mouth, and attaching teeth to it in some way or other, is so simple that any quack can acquire a knowledge of it in a few weeks and start out as a dentist.

And dental education among the people being at such a low stand, the rubber charlatan can always find numbers that eagerly accept his offer to pull out all their teeth and insert new ones at about the cost of shoeing a horse decently. But the best qualities of rubber, in the hands of good dentists, often subserve a useful purpose, where the best teeth are selected with judgment, fitted with care, and all the skill possible is put upon the work. In attaching teeth to rubber by means of gold supports or block teeth by rubber to gold plates, and in various other combinations of gold and rubber, there is room for great display of talent; but the dentist must be fairly remunerated for such work. Rubber for dental purposes is of various colors, white, brown, red, black, pink, etc. Black is the strongest, but very few can be persuaded to take it. Red is the color generally used as it is less objectionable than black and stronger than pink. But pink rubber is preferable when properly strengthened with gold, or when used as a coating over red rubber at the more exposed portions of the plate; by hardening at the right temperature and by certain means employed afterward, it can be made to approach gum-color so nearly as to escape detection in most cases.

PIVOT TEETH.

There is no artificial substitute that imitates nature so completely and, in favorable cases, produces so little discomfort to the patient. A pivot tooth consists of an artificial crown, in which there is a hole which comes opposite that in the center of the natural root; the root is filed off even with the gum, or a trifle below, the canal is enlarged, and the crown is fitted to it and ingrafted upon it by means of a pivot of wood or metal. The six front roots above and below, especially the former, are the only ones upon which it is advisable to ingraft pivot teeth. The roots should be solid and free from disease. As the requisite drilling and filing sometimes excites peridental inflammation, it is generally advisable to extend the operation through several sittings, and then to have a temporary pivot fitted rather loosely for a few days.

Well-seasoned hickory is generally used for permanent pivots, but commonly they have to be changed every few years at furthest; besides, teeth so inserted are not so cleanly on account of the insinuation of fluids and particles of food into the space between crown and root. The better, but more expensive way, is to have a gold tube inserted into the root, into which a gold pivot extending from the crown, fits tightly enough to retain it in position, but not so firmly as to prevent the frequent removal of it for the purpose of cleaning.

Pivot teeth in the mouths of very careful people sometimes last a great many years without injurious effects; but generally they are worn much too long by those that hold on to them after the roots decay, become loose, or have abscesses formed at the extremities, regardless of bad breath, inflamed gums, and the injury to the other teeth by vitiated fluids.

REPLANTING, ETC.

Numerous cases have been recorded in which natural teeth removed by accident or mistake have been replaced in their sockets, and have grown firm in their places again. Encouraged by these instances of tolerance on the part of nature, it has become a common practice with some dentists to experiment by replanting extracted teeth, not too badly decayed, which have refused to submit to treatment, or which the patients would not have treated.

Success attends the operation frequently enough to justify the trial, and it would be performed much oftener were it not that many patients object, thinking that there would be a recurrence of their troubles if the offending member should be replaced. This is not a valid objection, at least as far as any present trouble is concerned, for if the forbearance of nature is not secured, the tooth may be very easily extracted again, generally by the fingers of the patient. Teeth affected with decay and abscess have been extracted, and after the sac has been cut off and the decayed place filled, have been replaced, afterward doing good service.

Operations still more singular have been successful. Dr. Garretson, of Philadelphia, gives the following case:

"I once, as an experiment, replaced in the mouth a central incisor tooth, which had been extracted twelve hours before, and although it had been carried in the pocket, enveloped in the usual collection of dust, tobacco, keys, knife, etc., the whole intervening time, I kept it in its socket until the parts became reconciled. Many years have since passed, and it seemed to me, when last I saw it, about as useful as in its palmiest days."

In my own practice I recently had the following case: A youth having been kicked in the face by a horse a few days before, was brought to me with one of his upper incisors broken entirely off at the margin of the gum. As an experiment, I extracted the root, joined the crown to it by a gold pivot and Guillois' cement, and three hours afterward replaced it into its socket. No trouble of any kind followed, and now after a lapse of four months, the tooth is as firm and useful as any in the mouth.

DEFECTS OF THE PALATE.

FROM malformation, accident, or disease, various defects of the palate may result, which interfere to a less or greater extent with mastication, swallowing, speech and comfort.

The inconvenience may at times be so great as to take away all pleasure of life until it is remedied. There may be a simple perforation of the palate only, which the patient readily learns to close by some home-made appliance; or a large portion of the palate and bones may be missing, requiring the most complicated apparatus.

It would be consuming space unnecessarily to mention the different kinds of palatine defects, and the method of remedying each, as the cases are generally so urgent that patients need no solicitation to avail themselves of the best surgical or dental skill. Suffice it to say that by the operation of staphyloraphy, by the insertion of obturators to close openings, or artificial palates to restore lost portions, the majority of palatine defects may be perfectly cured, or much improved. The operation of staphyloraphy consists in paring the borders of the cleft palate, stitching the raw edges together, and trusting to nature to unite them. The adaptation of obturators and artificial palates, requires more ingenuity and skillful workmanship than any other branch of mechanical dentistry.

QUACKERY.

THE American people have long enjoyed the unenviable reputation of being the most easily humbugged of any nation in the world. In no other country do cheap auctions, dollar stores, traveling impostors, catch-penny advertisements, quack doctors, etc., find so many dupes.

But in nothing is this trait exhibited to such a remarkable degree as in the love the people have for "cheap dentistry." On this account, many good men who have striven hard to elevate the profession, and to cultivate the appreciation of the people, have retired in disgust, and many more would do likewise if opportunities should offer for them to gain a better livelihood in some other way.

A still larger number, equally disgusted, yet love their profession so dearly that they cling to it, hoping for the day to come when the scales shall fall from the eyes of the people, although they can not but see that dental quackery becomes more rampant from day to day. Thousands of persons that would scornfully refuse the attendance of a quack physician, or who would be ashamed to wear imitation jewelry or cheap clothing, think it no disgrace to patronize the lowest dental charlatan.

Numbers of people that spend their thousands in their summer travels, horses, carriages and diamonds,

> " And sacrifice to dress,
> Till household joys and comforts cease,"

become strangely economical in their dental expenditures.

This state of affairs is to be attributed mainly to two causes—the lack of that dental information that I have endeavored to lay before my readers in the preceding pages of this volume, and the failure to discern the distinguishing marks between the true profession of dentistry and dental empiricism.

With a few remarks upon the latter and some kindred subjects, I shall conclude.

DENTAL QUALIFICATIONS.

WEBSTER defines a quack to be "one who boastfully pretends to knowledge not possessed; an ignorant and pretentious practitioner in any branch of knowledge." In dentistry the meaning of the term is extended to embrace those that have not served the term of pupilage and tuition that is required before they are deemed worthy of college diplomas, together with those, still lower in reputation, who, having graduated, are unwilling to labor for respect and reputable patronage, and disgrace their *Alma Mater*, and detract from the dignity of the profession by resorting to cheap advertisements and unprofessional trickery. What a state of society is that when intelligent people in an enlightened country, lost to all appreciation of one of nature's most valuable gifts, cast their pearls before swine by patronizing the laboratory student of a few weeks' experience, who flaunts his banners proclaiming "cheap dentistry," rather than pay a little more for the services of the worthy practitioner who has spent years of his life and much of his means in properly qualifying himself! When a man makes a quack dentist of himself, he could not by words more plainly express the fact that he is not qualified to command a first-class patronage. If he could, he would certainly prefer it, but knowing his inability, his only hope is to get up an extensive practice among the ignorant, poor and penurious.

A dental diploma does not of itself, however, make a competent dentist; but it shows that he has appreciated the importance of his calling enough to place himself in the proper position for acquiring the requisite knowledge, and it is a letter of introduction to public notice from an experienced faculty, asserting that the graduate is master of the theory of dentistry, and has passed a creditable examination. The start being right, the most of the requisite knowledge and skill is to be acquired by study and experience afterward. No professional men are more exposed to criticism than dentists, and people are constantly taking them to task for failings that often have nothing to do with their competency. Some prefer an old man to a younger one on account of his greater experience; others prefer the latter because they think that the sight of the former is not so good, or that he is an old fogy, or that he has become too independent or indifferent. Other things being equal, a dentist ought to improve as he grows older, within certain limits; but some men can learn more in five years than others can in a lifetime.

One dentist may make so many grammatical errors, mispronounce so many words of his own language, and murder his Latin so extensively, that he causes his refined and educated patients to leave him in disgust, and yet he may be a skillful operator and an excellent mechanic. His manner may be harsh, his dress may be out of style, he may hold opposite political and religious views, he may be of very homely appearance, he may be poorly educated in general matters, and a poor conversationalist, and yet his dental work may be of the best quality. But no dentist is worthy of reputable patronage that is not master of his profession, a gentleman in his manners, cleanly about his office, free from demoralizing habits, honest in his dealings with his patients, and of good character; while he may reasonably expect to be more and more successful, the more nearly he meets the requirements of modern, refined, intellectual and religious society.

ADVERTISING, ETC.

The prevailing feeling among dentists of repute in regard to dental advertisements is about the same as that expressed in the Code of Dental Ethics:

"It is unprofessional to resort to public advertisements, cards, handbills, posters, or signs, calling attention to peculiar styles of work, lowness of prices, special modes of operating; or to claim superiority over neighboring practitioners; to publish reports of cases or certificates in the public prints; to go from house to house to solicit or perform operations; to circulate or recommend nostrums; or to perform any other similar acts."

No dentist is ever censured for putting up neat signs with his name and title, or for issuing any number of similar cards or advertisements to call attention to his place of business, and invite the public patronage; but how far he can transgress these bounds and maintain his professional standing, has been a subject of much discussion. On the one hand, those who after years of effort have established a large practice, are often, doubtless, too stringent; while, on the other, those who have not been successful, or those who are just beginning to practice, are often too liberal in their views. In many cases, where the striving dentist keeps anywhere near the bounds of propriety, more leniency ought to be exercised by his professional brethren; for domestic wants, unpaid bills and empty pockets are strong incentives for a man to do many things to court patronage, that he would scorn to do in better circumstances. But when a man openly disregards all claims of professional decorum, and resorts to paid puffs, advertisements of cheap rates, or work superior to that of others, he becomes a quack, no matter what his standing may have been previously.

CHARGES.

There is such a wide range between the fees asked by different dentists, that confusion often results among patients in estimating what is and what is not an equivalent for prices paid. There are two extremes—that of extortion on one side, and that of empiricism on the other. It seems to me that the fair dentist ought to avoid both extremes, and require only a reasonable remuneration; but every one has a right to place his own estimate upon his services, provided that the patient is informed of the price before the work is done. It is certainly poor policy for a dentist to overcharge his patient because he knows that he possesses abundant means; it is like killing the goose that laid the golden egg. It is a question to be decided by one's own conscience, whether or not it is right for a professional man, standing as a public benefactor, to exact such fees that the wealthy alone can secure his services. One thing is certain, however, that a dentist whose charges are high, is rarely guilty of doing poor work, and the latter is a more disgraceful accusation than the former.

The same truth, that a dentist has a right to set his own value upon his services, holds good even in the business of the charlatan. If he finds his duties so pleasing to his tastes that he considers five or ten dollars, and the inhalation of a fetid breath, a sufficient remuneration for a protracted operation upon a diseased mouth, extracting old roots and inserting a set of his inimitable teeth, well and good,—no one envies him his job.

WARRANTIES.

The most reputable practitioners of dentistry never warrant their work; quacks, without a dollar in their pockets, and whose promises are worth even less, will guarantee against all accidents, possible and impossible, for all time to come. It is deemed unprofessional to give warranties. In taking this stand it is intended to teach the people that dentistry is a branch of medicine just as much as is the profession of the oculist or the aurist, and that its practitioners are entitled to the same respect.

What person afflicted with a disease of the eye or ear, would insult his physician by asking him to warrant that he should be cured and should remain so? No one engaged in any business or profession, has as much responsibility expected of him as the dentist.

When persons are sick they send for a physician in whom they have confidence, ask no guarantees, and trust altogether to his honor and professional reputation. If after a certain length of time he fails to do them any good, they may dismiss him and send for another; yet they pay him for every visit without grumbling, just as if they had recovered under his care. The lawyer receives pay for his services, whether he loses or gains his suit.

People buy watches and jewelry that are subjected to far easier usage than the teeth are, and though they break again and again, they expect to pay for repairing. A fine vehicle bought to-day, may have a wheel knocked off to-morrow, and an extra charge is made for repairing. The shoemaker gets paid for patching, and the tailor for mending.

Even the works of nature give way; trees blow down, and living things die unexpectedly, but the work of the dentist is often expected to be infallible. It is not an uncommon thing for a person to wear a set for five or ten years with every satisfaction, and then if a tooth comes off, demand that it shall be put on again without charge. Others, with mouths so unfavorable that it is impossible to adapt a set of teeth to them, although the dentist tries again and again to do it, generously offer not to trouble him any more if he will refund their money.

To those that are acquainted with the good professional standing of a dentist, his promise to serve them to the best of his capacity should be enough.

To transient patients that know nothing of his reputation, there is nothing unprofessional in warranting that the materials used shall be of the quality contracted for, and that he and his assistants will exert themselves to the best of their ability to make good all representations. But it is unprofessional and one-sided for a dentist to warrant fillings to last a certain number of years for those that may make no effort to preserve them, or to warrant artificial sets of teeth not to break for those that may fracture them by the roughest usage, or by accident, and then attempt to impose upon the dentist by asserting that they broke without any strain whatever. Every dentist knows that it is to his interest to do all he can, consistently with duty, to satisfy his patients; and there are very few practitioners indeed, that will not go to the full limit of their obligations in re-filling, re-inserting plates, or in correcting any errors, to retain their patients. But if any misunderstanding as to the dentist's responsibility should arise, the patient should not make the dental office the scene of unpleasant wrangling, but should exercise his liberty of leaving his dentist just as he would a physician that treated him unsuccessfully.

DENTAL HARMONY.

Dentists, like other professional men, have their piques, cliques, jealousies, disputes and prejudices, which, however much they may be deprecated, can hardly be wondered at as long as human nature is what it is, and different schools, sectional peculiarities, and individual rivalries exist. Those animated discussions that take place at dental societies and conventions, and in the different periodicals, doubtless result in great good by eliciting the various views of the combatants, and starting an energy of thought that would not be aroused in any other way.

But when the dentists of any one locality can not agree among themselves, and descend to petty quarrels and personal envy and abuse, they certainly thereby much hinder the advancement of the profession; for its progress depending upon the estimation of the people, it is not natural that they can have the greatest respect for those that on account of private envy, or mercenary motives, endeavor to injure one another.

Travelers through various sections of the country have noticed great difference in the amount of harmonious feeling existing among dentists. In some locations, the dentists, bound by the strongest bonds of fraternal feeling, crowd their offices together in the same building, meet often in social intercourse, shield one another's faults, attend to one another's practices during absence, and extend the hand of welcome to all worthy incoming practitioners. In other places, they scatter their offices far apart, seldom or never hold meetings, make mole-hill failings into mountain faults, would rather drop at their chairs than trust their practices to one another, and turn the cold shoulder to those that are striving to advance themselves, till they are driven away from the place, or become quacks through desperation.

No honorable dentist, however, can refrain from treating the charlatan as he deserves, for such a man is the avowed enemy of the profession, and makes it his whole object to degrade it. And all dentists being open to public criticism, if they depart so far from propriety in their professional labors or social relations as to make their faults notorious, their most forgiving brethren can not help being occasionally drawn into conversations that may be disparaging to them.

In placing this volume before the public, I would only say in conclusion, that if my endeavor to give the people useful information concerning the teeth, and to call attention to various subjects of mutual interest to the dentist and the public, have been successful in awakening a better appreciation of the teeth and of the profession that makes the preservation of them a specialty, I am abundantly rewarded.

But if I have failed in my object, and the reader feels like saying:

'I pray thee, cease thy counsel,
Which falls into my ears as profitless
As water in a sieve,"

I shall at least take comfort in thinking with Byron:

" 'Tis pleasant sure to see one's name in print;
A book's a book, although there's nothing in 't."

INDEX.

	PAGE.
Abrasion of the teeth	169
Abscess, alveolar	150
Acids, effects upon the teeth	83
Advertising, etc	262
Alloys, fusible	101
Aluminum plates	247
Alveolar abscess	150
Amalgam	101
Anæsthesia	201
Anæsthetics, local and general	200
relative safety of	220
Antrum, diseases of the	172
Arsenic, for devitalizing the pulp, and the dangers of	145
Artificial teeth	233
preparation of the mouth for	233
Atrophy	167
Battery, electro-galvanic	201
Bleaching discolored teeth	131
Bleeding, and how to control it	195
Brushes for the teeth	228
Capping exposed nerves	113
Caries	77
causes of	82
prevention of	89
Cementum, description of	70
exposed	157
Charges for dental services	263
Charlatanism	258
Cheoplastic metal	246
Clasp plates	240
Cleaning the teeth	89
Cleft palate, etc	256
Coffer dam rubber	130
Continuous gum plates	242
Creasote, care in the use of	143
Crowded wisdom-teeth	64
Crusta petrosa, description of	70

	PAGE.
Decay	77
causes of	82
prevention of	89
Decomposition in the pulp cavity	153
Dental harmony	266
Dental pulp, description of	70
Dentifrices	226
Dentine, description of	69
Dentine, sensitive	109
remedies for	111
Dentistry, history of	13
Dentition, first	40
troubles of	43
second	60
troubles of	64
third	183
Denudation of the teeth	171
Destroying the nerve	144
Discolored teeth	131, 158
Diseases of first dentition	46
Dislocation of the jaw	198
Empiricism	258
Enamel, description of the	67
Eruption of the permanent teeth	60
of the temporary teeth	40
Ether spray	201
Exostosis	155
Exposed nerves, capping of	113
Extracting	189
dangers of	190
difficulties of	192
during pregnancy	195
File, the use of the	125, 128
Filling the teeth	93
Filling roots	117
First dentition, diseases of	46
lancing the gums during	49
mortality during	44

	PAGE.
Formation of the teeth	34
Food in relation to the teeth	21
Fungous gum	155
pulp	154
Fusible alloys	101
Galvanic battery	201
Gas, nitrous oxide	203
safety of	219
Gold fillings	98
plates	244
Guarantees	264
Guillois' cement	102
Gum-boils	150
Gums, diseased, prescriptions for	179, 180
Gums, inflammation of	177
Gutta percha	102
Harmony among dentists	266
Hemorrhage	195
treatment of	196
Hill's stopping	102
History of dentistry	13
Inflammation of the gums	177
Irregularity of the teeth	71
Irritation of the pulp	140
Jaw, dislocation of the	198
Key instrument for extracting	191
Lancing the gums	49, 194
method of	53
Laughing gas	203
safety of	219
Lime, phosphate of	23
Magnified tooth, plate of	68
Mallet filling	122
Maxillary sinus, diseases of the	172
Milk	26
adulterations of	28
Mineral plates	244
Molars, first permanent	62
Mortality during first dentition	44
Mouth, preparation of the, for artificial teeth	236
Mouth-washes	179, 228
Necrosis	158
Neuralgia	160
Nitrous oxide	203
dangers of	223
experiments with	212
how to inhale	206
generation of	204
safety of	219

	PAGE.
Odontalgia	138
different forms of	139
treatment of	142
Origin of the teeth	31
Os-artificiel	162
Osseous union of the teeth	188
Oxy-chloride of zinc	102
Palate, defects of the	256
Periodontitis	147
Permanent first molars	62
teeth	59
teeth, description of	66
Phosphate of lime	23
Pivot teeth	253
Plate of magnified tooth	68
of the permanent teeth	61
of the temporary teeth	41
Plates, aluminum	247
cheoplastic	246
clasp	240
continuous gum	242
gold	244
mineral	244
rose-pearl	248
rubber	250
silver	246
suction	240
temporary	238
Plugging	93
Porcelain teeth	241
Powders for the teeth	227
Pregnancy, toothache of	193
Preservation of the temporary teeth	55
Prevention of decay	89
Pulp, decomposition of the	153
description of the	70
devitalization of the	144
fungous	154
irritation	140
nodules	146
Quackery	258
Qualifications of the dentist	259
Ranula	176
Regulating	74
Replanting teeth	234
Rhigolene	201
Root filling	117
Roots, extraction of	193
preservation of	121
"Rose-pearl"	248
Rubber dam	130
plates	250
rings in regulating	76

	PAGE.
Salivary calculus	133
effects of	136
removal of	137
ducts, closure of the	176
Second dentition, troubles of	64
Sensitive dentine	109
remedies for	111
Separating	127
Silver plates	246
Spray of ether	201
Suction plates	240
Sugar	29
Supernumerary teeth	186
Sympathetic pain	160
Tartar	133
effects of	136
removal of	137
Teeth, brushes for the	228
classes of	80
artificial	233
artificial, preparation of the mouth for	236
effects of acids, etc., upon the	83
eruption of the temporary	40
eruption of the permanent	60
food in relation to the	21
how to clean the	89
irregularity of the	71
origin and formation of	34
permanent	59
permanent, description of the	66

	PAGE.
Teeth, permanent, plate of the	61
pivot	253
porcelain	241
powders	227
supernumerary	186
Temporary plates	238
teeth, plate of the	41
teeth, preservation of the	55
Third dentition	183
Tin foil	101
Tobacco, effects of	229
Toothache	133
different forms of	139
treatment of	142
of children	146
prescription for	146
Tooth-key	191
Tooth-marks	167
Troubles of first dentition	43
of second dentition	64
Tumors of the mouth	180
United teeth	188
Vulcanized rubber plates	250
Warranties	264
Washes for the mouth	179, 224
Wearing away of the teeth	169
Wedging	128
Wet-nurse	27
White filling	102
Wisdom-teeth, crowded	64

www.ingramcontent.com/pod-product-compliance
Lightning Source LLC
Chambersburg PA
CBHW032002230426
43672CB00010B/2243